Praise for It's Time for a PAUSE

Dr Renata's book should be read by all midlife women, from when the first symptoms of menopause appear, to when they end, and beyond. I had so much pleasure reading this book. She makes it easy to understand, the things many women experience, and shares what the safest approaches are for treatment of several of the symptoms. Being a breast cancer survivor and having experience in my medical practice with hormone replacement, I understand that hormonal therapy may not be appropriate for every woman. Dr Renata's approach offers alternative treatment options, including proper diet, supplements, exercises, and support groups. I will recommend this book to all my patients.

Maria Briones, MD, medical director Briones Weight Loss Clinic, Mount Kisco, NY

If you're a woman, you must read *It's Time for a PAUSE*. From the very first paragraph, you will feel like you're not alone anymore in your menopausal, hormonal roller-coaster journey. Dr. Renata speaks right to your heart, and I found myself nodding the entire time as she shared her own menopausal journey and all the ups and downs associated with it. There is naivety and a lack of information from much of the medical community. Not only does Dr. Renata make you feel like you are part of an empowered female community, but she also gives simple and effective tools and strategies to implement to ease the symptoms of menopause. The message here is, you don't have to give up and give in!

Dr. Amie Hornaman, "The Thyroid Fixer"
nutritionist, founder of the Institute for Thyroid
and Hormone Optimization

It's Time for a PAUSE is a gift to women looking for a warm, knowledgeable source to guide them through menopause. Dr. Shiloah supports women through this powerful journey with an extensive clinical background paired with her signature grace and wisdom, so readers know they're not alone.

Dr. Jessica Titchenal, DCN, MS, CNS, CN,
intuitive medium, and health coach

IT'S TIME FOR A PAUSE

It's not often you find someone in your life who is a friend, mentor, and colleague rolled into one, but that's what Dr. Renata Shiloah is to me. Additionally, she and I seem to be living parallel lives, which is why I was so excited to read an early copy of her book, *It's Time for a Pause*. I recently entered into a new chapter (no pun intended) of my life called menopause and was struggling to make sense of the changes happening within me. Dr. Renata combines her personal and professional insights, along with tangible takeaways—in the form of journal pages, activities, and reflective poetry through the book—to help you navigate a seemingly complex situation into a more manageable one.

Dina R. D'Alessandro, MS, RDN, CDN
(she/her), founder and chief executive life-changer at DishWithDina

Dr. Renata has the ability to relate to you so you may find self-confidence again. She wants to know and understand you to really help you succeed in your goals and overcome your challenges. She treats her patients as equals. I can't even put into words how much she has helped me.

Diana, patient

Dr. Renata is understanding, compassionate, helpful, patient, and just a great encouraging guide through your wellness journey. She was our dietician but also our therapist and friend. She was there for us and just so loving and welcoming. I know there are amazing dieticians out there, but Dr. Renata treats us like we were part of her family.

Norma, patient

Dr. Renata has always encouraged me to go further, do better and it's just the faith she has in me when sometimes I don't even see it in myself. She's the best, I don't know anyone else that cares about everyone that goes there. She always makes time for her patients. I can call her right now and say I need to speak to her, and she will listen and give me the best advice. She just supports me in every part of my life. I will always remember Dr. Renata's positive attitude, compassion, humbleness and how wise she is.

Angelica, patient

IT'S TIME FOR A PAUSE

How to Fight Back Against Menopause,
Naturally Reduce Symptoms, and
Feel Like Yourself Again

DR. RENATA SHILOAH

DCN, MS, RD, CDN, RYT, CMT

Disclaimer
The information contained in this book *It's Time for a PAUSE,* is provided for educational purposes only. It is not meant to replace professional medical advice, diagnosis, or treatment. Any attempt to diagnose and or treat a medical condition should be done under the guidance of a medical doctor. It is recommended to consult with a medical doctor before using any information, idea, recipe, or products discussed in this book, including within the yoga and meditation chapter. Neither the authors nor the publisher shall be liable or responsible for any loss or adverse effects allegedly resulting from any information or suggestions in this book. While every effort has been made to ensure the accuracy of the information presented in this book, neither the authors nor the publisher assumes any responsibility for errors. References are provided for information purposes only and do not constitute endorsement of any websites or other sources. Readers should be aware that the information in the websites, sources, and references listed in this book may change over time.

ISBN: 9798218134747 (Paperback)

Front cover image by Whitney Photography
Makeup for cover image by Melora Yaru
Cover design and interior formatting by Hannah Linder
Designs
Editing by vocem LLC
www.nutritionist4u.com

To my dear mother, Jarmila, who was my best friend. We called her Baji, a nickname for grandma, of which she was the best. She bravely rode through her menopause journey in silence.

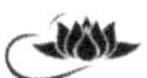

To my dear daughter, Daniella, and my miraculous granddaughter, Lucy: may you never experience significant menopausal symptoms during your menopause journeys. I love you both.

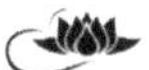

To my husband, Eli, and my four amazing son's—Micky, Teddy, Jonathan, and Benjamin. Thank you for putting up with me during my darkest times on my menopause journey.

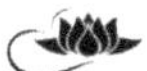

A very heartfelt dedication to Danielle and Laura, two special women who left us too soon.

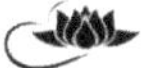

Finally, this book is dedicated to all the midlife women suffering needlessly, the women who feel as if they are losing their minds. You are not alone on this transitional midlife journey. You do not have to stay or become "broken" in midlife. You can naturally heal your body and mind and once again live the life you deserve!

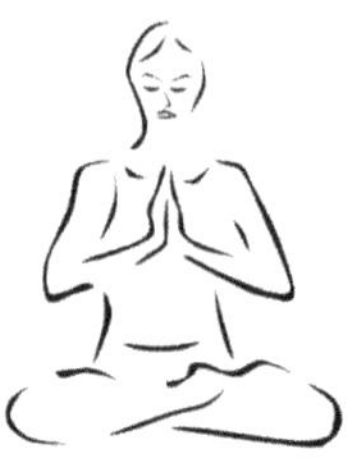

Contents

Foreword

Every woman who experiences menopause will encounter some surprises. It's common to feel surprised about your surprises too. Such is midlife. Menopause is just one more unexpected eye-opener!

As a master life coach, midlife mentor, podcast host, and author, I hear this all the time. Being a midlife coach is my second career, starting in 2014. Before this, I worked in the field of health education and health promotion for twenty-seven years.

It was my work as a midlife coach that brought Renata and me together. We've known each other since 2020, and she's an active, contributive member of my Women in the Middle® community.

"Women in the Middle" is the name I came up with for my coaching work with midlife women, especially the fifty-plus category. I thought "women in the middle" described this midlife phase of a woman's life perfectly. Midlife women are in the middle of a variety of complex transitions, including the empty nest, their aging bodies, their aging mindsets, changing relationships, plans for retirement, milestone birthdays, long-term careers, caring for parents, long-term marriages, a newfound sensitivity to wasting time, and, of course, menopause.

Menopause is a topic that women in the middle tend to grapple with because, like many other midlife topics, there is a lack of awareness about the impact menopause can have, creating confusion and unhappiness. One common goal that clients, the women in my community, and the listeners of my podcast share is the desire for more clarity so they don't have regrets about what they didn't do, didn't try, or didn't say. A lack of awareness leads to a lack of clarity. This all creates real problems in midlife when you're particularly sensitive to wasting valuable time. You don't feel empowered; instead, you feel like you're at the mercy of something you have no control over.

Dr. Renata knew this about the women in her community too. She also knew that she had a message that had to get out. She forged an ability to help women empower themselves to fight back and feel like themselves again.

Her combination of evidence-based information and a holistic approach, with her compassionate voice, creates a much-needed message in this space. In her own words, *"It's Time for a PAUSE* is a collection of safe and scientifically-proven, integrative healing therapies to aid with menopausal symptom relief."* She presents an easy-to-understand road map forward when you don't even recognize yourself anymore.

Dr. Renata includes several relatable examples. She shares her personal story, including some of her specific thoughts about the things she was going through on her menopausal journey. As a mindset coach, I appreciate her transparency. For example, one of her powerful thoughts was, "I am worthy and will not allow anything to stand in the way of the happiness I deserve," which emphasizes the importance of creating intentional thoughts and an intentional mindset to rely on, even when you need to remind yourself.

It's Time for a PAUSE is a powerful yet easily digestible book, full of compassion, guidance, and lessons to guide you through a potentially challenging and confusing part of your life as a woman. Thankfully, we have Dr. Renata's experience and love to help us navigate our way through it. This book feels like a hug!

Suzy Rosenstein, MA, master coach, midlife mentor, host of Women in the Middle® Midlife Podcast

The Stranger Inside Me

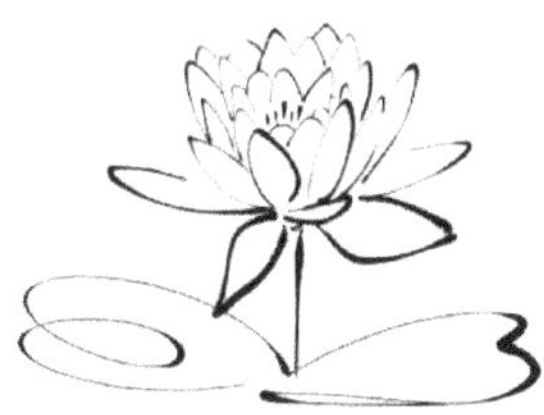

I feel a stranger lurking deep inside my mind, yet
this person is so very hard to find.
She experiences tragedy, she experiences pain.
it is really a shame.

Why can't she be the person who is not afraid of dark,
not afraid of light, not afraid of people, and not afraid to
fight.

This stranger is a stranger that is stranger than them all,
every time I see her, she is stranger than before.
Why can't she go away?
I pray, I pray, I pray.

She doesn't listen, I feel that she is here,
throughout eternity, seasons, and the years.

*I have to learn to love her, because she will never die,
you see, she is not she for she is I.*

~ Dr. Renata

Preface

I wrote this book for you—the midlife woman living the life I did before I put the information from this book into play in my own life. For you, the woman suffering needlessly like I was, *was* being the magic word! Wouldn't it be great if you could tell *your* story and use the word *was*? As women, we face numerous challenges during our lives, some harder to deal with than others. We come across countless obstacles in our families, work, responsibilities, and a lack of knowledge and time. Ask yourself, "What is my biggest obstacle at this moment?" No matter what the answer is, get into the mindset that you *can* and *will* make a change for the better and live the life you deserve by following the simple steps I've outlined in this book.

It's Time for a PAUSE holds the keys to easing or even eliminating your menopausal symptoms. Before you spend thousands of dollars on over-the-counter supplements or commit to optional prescription medications, which may cause side effects worse than your menopausal symptoms, read this book. I, like you, experienced years filled with needless symptoms, such as weight gain, bloating, brain fog, painful joints, and irritability —just to name a few. If I had read a book like this one before I felt "broken," I would have saved myself years of unnecessary suffering and thousands of dollars.

One note: Be sure to read this book from cover to cover. I am confident we will touch on your specific symptom(s) and you'll understand what your body is telling you, what may have caused it, and what can help alleviate or eliminate it. You will find a clear explanation for each common menopausal symptom, a list of therapeutic foods, gentle yoga moves, and a meditation to aid with quick relief so you can feel like yourself again.

You are not alone. I've included stories from women just like you, sharing about their triumphs over the menopausal battle.

It's Time for a PAUSE is a collection of safe and scientifically proven integrative healing therapies to aid with menopausal symptom relief. I've based the information inside on a holistic, integrative approach to focus on the causes, rather than the symptoms themselves. These are unlike conventional methods, which solely treat symptoms, such as prescribing medication for joint pain. When the effects of the pain medication wear off, the joint discomfort returns—perhaps even more intensely. Focusing on the cause of menopausal symptoms and using a healthy diet and integrative healing practices are the keys to menopause relief.

Integrative therapies, such as yoga and meditation, have been proven to relieve the common symptoms women experience during the menopausal years and have been practiced by women for thousands of years, even before people understood the science behind it.[1] Medical doctors now combine conventional therapies with alternative ones. That's why I offer scientific facts based on innovative research on integrative therapies' effects on menopausal symptoms. Modern women need options other than simple conventional treatments, like hormone replacement and medications. Yoga and meditation aid women with reconnecting with their inner selves. These practices can assist with discovering from where symptoms stem, therefore making recovery easier. Taking a breath and relaxing our minds help to bring us into the present moment, which is where healing begins.[2]

It's Time for a PAUSE is for you—whether you're anxious about making changes or eager to make changes. The woman ready to get back her life, the woman who has never practiced yoga or meditation, and the woman who tried and gave up all need this book. I can't promise that you'll feel twenty-five again, but I do promise you will be in your forties, fifties, and beyond, feeling fabulous, with just a few tweaks to your daily habits! It's never too late to make changes.

It's Time for a PAUSE has been written from a professional and personal perspective and is meant to help women reverse the overwhelming state menopause can cause physically, emotionally, and mentally. It offers the most cost-effective approach to reclaiming and sustaining who you really are.

This book is not meant to replace conventional medicine; it is intended to supplement and aid other options to provide positive results. My hope is to make the process of relief from menopausal symptoms a pleasant journey back to your true self. Take action, don't just dream about getting your life back . . . or when you wake up, life will have passed you by. Let's dive in!

I Slumber in the Sky

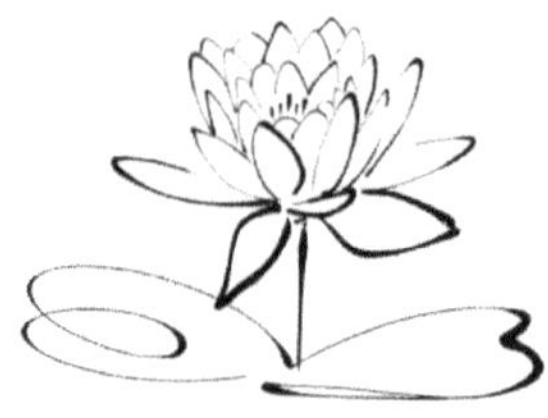

I slumber and stare at the sky
I dream in clouds, as I pray and cry
I endlessly dream, as living passes me by
My dreams are real, they are what I feel
I dream of happy times, times without pain

Times when my life, wasn't insane

Why am I dreaming, why am I here?

Why can't I float away, into the atmosphere?
I'll never wake up; I'll never be me
I'll never know what could be.
In my dreams, I have been here and there
In my dreams, I have been everywhere
I dream of riches, I dream of gold
I dream that my life, in front of me, will unfold

I cannot stay asleep forever, for one day
I will wake up and say,
Good I did not dream my life away

~ Dr. Renata

Introduction

Thousands of women reach menopause every day in the United States, which equates to over two million per year. Menopause is defined by most dictionaries as the end of a woman's menstrual cycle. On average, this occurs in women between the ages of forty and fifty-five. Menopause results in a decrease in hormones, causing ovarian follicular function decline. The official stage of menopause begins when the menstrual cycle stops for a full twelve months. However, menopausal symptoms, such as hot flashes, mood swings, bloating, weight gain, insomnia, and more, start years earlier, which is referred to as perimenopause. On average, perimenopause lasts for seven to fourteen years, depending on factors, such as lifestyle, age at onset, and race and ethnicity. (*What Is Menopause? | National Institute on Aging,* n.d.).

When I was younger, I had no idea what menopause would be like because that season of life never occurred to me. Not even when I started my period or gave birth to my first child. I don't think I had ever used the *"M* word" before going through the "change of life" myself. Isn't it amazing how rapidly things change?

When I was twelve years old, I couldn't wait to be thirteen so I could be an official teenager. When I was thirteen, I couldn't wait to be sixteen so I could get my driver's license. When I was sixteen, I couldn't wait until I was eighteen so I could be classified as an adult. Then, I couldn't wait to be twenty-one.

When I reached age forty, I stopped wanting to rush time. I wanted to *pause* and stay forty forever, but that didn't happen. Birthday after birthday still came. Period after period. And then one day, my body started acting as if it had a mind of its own. I eventually discovered perimenopause was the culprit. Since you're reading this book, you're likely pre-menopausal or going through menopause, maybe having symptoms and wanting to get your body back under control so you can feel like yourself again. Well, guess what? You are not alone!

I'm Not Afraid

I'm not afraid of sorrow,
I'm not afraid of pain

I'm not afraid of happiness,
I'm not afraid of shame,

I'm not afraid of people,
I'm not afraid of change,

I'm not afraid of the ocean,
I'm not afraid of the sea,

I'm not afraid of you,
But I am afraid of me!

~ Dr. Renata

My Menopause Journey

My mother never spoke to me about menopause or anything that has to do with hormones. My mother was an old-fashioned, timid woman from Europe. My PMS (premenstrual syndrome) blew out of control in my early forties. I was at work one day and panicked, thinking I had some horrible disease when the symptoms of bloating, anxiety, brain fog, and cramping hit. I ran to my car for privacy and called my gynecologist (a male). Through tears, I told him about my symptoms, still believing I was dying.

My doctor paused for a minute, then said, "You are officially in perimenopause, which may last for ten or more years." I couldn't believe my ears . . . *ten* years or more?! *Has he lost his mind? Did I lose my mind? What am I going to do?* I was scared of what was to come. As a director of nutrition in a network of five outpatient clinics, I had to "look good" for patients; I had to feel fantastic and set a good example. Yet when I looked in the mirror, all I could do was cry. My confidence was gone, so I had to play the role of the person I used to be and unleash my waves of emotion in private.

I felt stressed each morning as I thought about the day ahead and the "acting" I had to do. I even bought a book, *Acting for the Non-Actor.* Depression and anxiety set in, but I was a pro at keeping them hidden. I lived with my dark secret hidden from the world for a few years.

One day, I decided I would not continue the dark journey. I made dietary changes and bought a book about running. I began to feel less depressed and my symptoms—the weight gain, bloating, brain fog, and aches and pains—improved. I joined a local running group and eventually, I was running thirty-five miles each week, segmented into three or four runs. I felt great, and it showed! My body transformed; I lost weight, felt happier, and my husband commented that my body looks like that of an athlete!

Unfortunately, when I took on a new position as the director of nutrition with a longer commute and greater job responsibilities, I stopped running. I felt the exhaustion of trying to maintain the exercise routine which no longer fit into my new schedule. Lo and behold, my symptoms returned with a vengeance. So I took on a new hobby—hot yoga—which I loved, but because of my work schedule, I only had the opportunity to go at night, which left me more exhausted the next morning.

When the COVID-19 pandemic hit, I stopped everything. No hot yoga, no activity at all, and most of my workday was spent sitting in front of a computer while working. My symptoms returned one by one.

The positive part of sitting was that it allowed me to *pause* and think about my journey, including everything I'd learned as a nutritionist and the countless people (including myself) I had assisted in finding relief.

Though I felt "broken," depressed, and sluggish and loathed what my body and mind had become once again, I stood up from my chair, walked over to the mirror (which had become my enemy), and promised myself that I would never feel that way again. I also made a commitment to share my *"pause"* formula for vibrancy, health, and happiness with all of the "broken" women who now suffer as I did.

Sixteen in Two Million

As mentioned earlier, two million women per year reach menopause.[1] While everyone's experience is different, there is one thing that remains constant: We all need a *PAUSE* to overcome our symptoms. To prove this, I interviewed sixteen women from diverse backgrounds and experiences and got the scoop on their menopause journeys. I have added a few of their stories in this book, and you can read more stories on my website. I was not surprised to find that though parts of their stories differ, they are all still similar. No matter where you come from, what your ethnicity is, or what values you hold, menopause is inevitable. As females, we are all on the same journey in life, but *how* we ride through the waves is what makes the difference.

Most of the women I interviewed felt isolated and alone in their journeys. Talking about their experiences during the interviews made them feel less alone and isolated. My hope is that this book will unite you with like-minded women who are on the same journey and help you remember that you are not alone.

The stories I share from these sixteen midlife women will likely resonate with you. To show you what I mean, here are a few quotes from the ladies related to their experiences on their menopause journeys:

- "I can say that maybe I'm a little short-tempered." ~Marisol
- "I wish someone had told me that it could be early in life. I believe stress aids in bringing it on earlier. I wish doctors offered more natural means; they pushed medications and hormones too quickly for me." ~Letty
- "The symptoms I experienced during menopause were hot flashes, anxiety, mood swings, insomnia, and night sweats. I will never forget how I had to change my nightgown at least two times every night because of my night sweats. It came to the point that I would have to sleep with a towel on my bed and pillow to absorb the sweat. Once I began going through the changes, I could relate to what other women went through but realized soon enough that not everyone shared the same experiences. My sisters,

for example, didn't have the same experience as me. Thankfully, I had friends who understood what I was going through. (They) quickly became my support group." ~Janet

Studies show that approximately 85 percent of women experience menopausal symptoms by the age of fifty-four (Suzuki et al., 2014); for most women, menopausal symptoms begin between the ages of forty and fifty-eight—and even earlier in life for some.

Through my research and interviews, I found there is consistent evidence showing that environment, as well as social interaction, can contribute to the intensity of symptoms, particularly mood swings, during the menopausal transition period. One main conclusion I determined from my research is nearly all menopausal women report that their quality of life significantly decreased. This has caused them increased emotional distress, depression, and anxiety, as well as symptoms related to body aches, bloating, and weight gain. Menopause can be a vicious cycle for most women.

Activity: The Menopause Questionnaire

There are over forty symptoms contributing to menopause. If your symptoms are troubling, you will benefit from this book in many ways. If they are not, this book may help you prevent future symptoms. Women experience a variety of symptoms caused by hormones that are involved with the menopausal phase. The key to relief is knowing how to successfully manage the changes inside your body during this stage of life. Use the below chart to check off which of the forty common menopausal symptoms you are experiencing or have experienced.

40 Common Menopausal Symptoms

Symptom	YES	NO
Anxiety		
Bloating		
Brain Fog		
Breast Soreness		
Brittle Nails		
Burning Mouth Syndrome		
Chills		
Cold Hands and Feet		
Concentration Difficulties		
Crying Spells		
Decreased Libido		
Depression		
Dry Skin		
Electric Shocks		
Fatigue		
Hair Loss		
Headaches		
Hot Flashes		
Increased Blood Pressure		
Increased Cholesterol		
Irregular Heartbeat		
Irritability		
Itching		
Joint Pain		
Loss of Breast Fullness		
Migraines		
Mood Swings		
Night Sweats		
Not Enjoying Life as Before		
Osteoporosis		
Panic Attacks		
Personality Changes		
Random Hives		
Slower Metabolism		
Trouble Sleeping		
Urinary Incontinence		
Urinary Urgency		
Vaginal Dryness		
Weight Gain		
Worsening of Allergies		

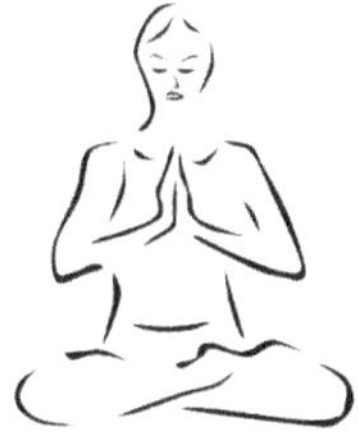

JOURNAL BREAK

A Time to *PAUSE* and Reflect

Now that we have gotten to know each other, and you have checked off your menopausal symptoms. I want you to journal about your thoughts and feelings and anything else you want to jot down related to your experience on your personal midlife journey. We will do this several times throughout the book.

____

____

____

____

____

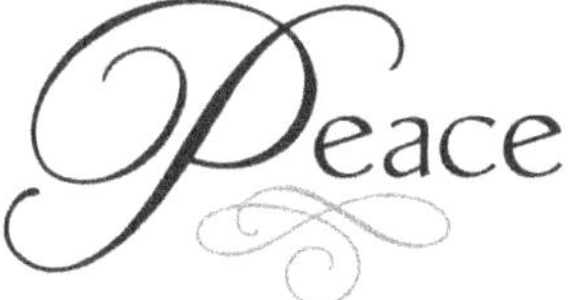

Chapter 1
HELLO, BEAUTIFUL

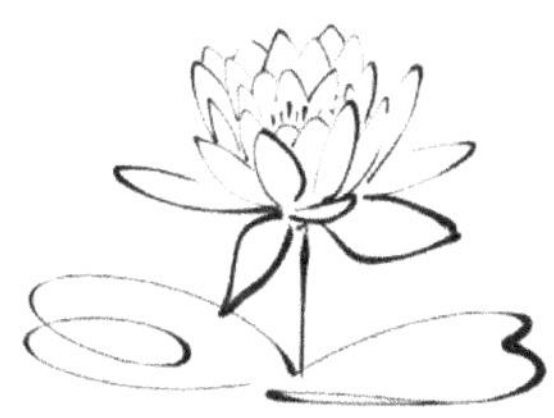

You Are Beautiful

You are beautiful, you are like the sun
You are beautiful because you are a unique one.
You are beautiful, you are a queen
You are beautiful inside out and in between.
You are beautiful, you have to admit
You are beautiful, and that is it!

~ Dr. Renata

Hello Beautiful,

You are beautiful inside and out. You have so much to give to the world. You have been born with a gift, making you unique and special. And you have a lot of talent.

No matter your age, I believe you'll identify with my story as well as the story of many other women who are gracefully transitioning to their new phase of life. If you feel alone, I am here to tell you that you're not. And if you feel like you've lost yourself, I am confident you will find yourself through these pages.

To the woman who feels all alone in this journey, I see you and am you. I understand how difficult it is for you to open up to others about your challenges. I'm guessing you're used to shouldering others' burdens and doing everything you can to assist them, but you seldom get much in return. You care about people so deeply that you don't want to be a burden to them, so you keep your worries to yourself and suffer in silence. Like I used to, maybe you put on a brave face and pretend to be OK so you can continue to assist and encourage others. You're terrifyingly skilled at faking contentment; no one sees anything except what you want them to see. This, however, isolates you, making you feel that aloneness. But know this: you don't have to go through this on your own.

To the woman who feels like you have lost yourself: I know you may be experiencing symptoms that are robbing you of your happiness and causing you to wish it would be over soon, but I am writing to tell you the wait is over. When I started going through the changes, I was miserable. I didn't feel like going anywhere with anyone, even though previously, I wanted to go out all the time. I was not happy with my body or myself, and I didn't even want to venture outside, into public! I dreaded invitations to weddings and became antisocial. I had to find myself all over again, and if you feel like that, I hope you learn some tips that will help you get back to enjoying life again too.

I have returned to activities and am loving every minute of them. The mind and body are connected. If you feel better in your body, you feel better emotionally and vice versa. You can fight back against menopause—naturally reducing symptoms and feeling like yourself again.

I see you and am you. So I have included re-sources, journal prompts, and activities inside these pages that will help you experience some relief, physically, mentally, and emotionally. How do I know? My journey through menopause was a rough one until I found the secret "PAUSE" for-mula, which turned me from a wilting rose into a beautiful Lotus flower.

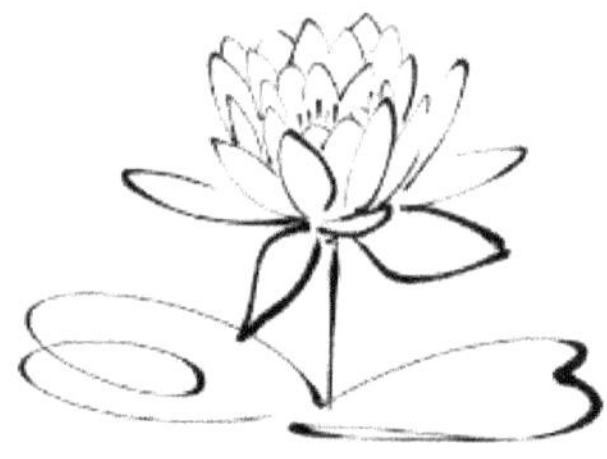

Like a Lotus Flower

Like a Lotus flower, you will . . .
Believe in yourself, and you will . . .
Like a Lotus flower, achieve the immeasurable.

Believe in yourself, and you will, like a Lotus flower,
select novel surroundings.

Believe in yourself, and you will, like a Lotus flower,
lessen difficulties associated with each resolution.

Believe in yourself, and you will, like a Lotus flower,

make the tough seem meek.

Believe in yourself, and you will, like a Lotus flower, relish the magnificence of the earth's creations.

Believe in yourself, and you will, like a Lotus flower, rise beyond your wildest expectations.

Believe in yourself, and you will, like a Lotus flower, discover talents hidden inside you.

Believe in yourself, and you will, like a Lotus flower, be purified as you continue to be exceptional and superior.

Believe in yourself, and you will, like a Lotus flower, acquire abilities and understanding from being.

Believe in yourself, and you will, like a Lotus flower, attain impossible dreams.

BELIEVE IN YOURSELF, like a Lotus flower, and YOU WILL!

~ Dr. Renata

I am excited to help guide you on your transitional journey into the next phase of life. Not only from a professional standpoint, but from my personal experience. I encourage you to stay positive, no matter what obstacles come your way. I want you to have a smooth ride, not a bumpy one like I did before I came to the realization that there is hope . . . and natural ways to find relief, other than conventional medicine. I got my life back and so can you!

Journal Prompt: A Letter of Expectation

Write a letter to yourself using the following prompts and journal pages (you can add or change the prompts as you feel necessary):

- Name your 3 most bothersome symptoms, the ones that haunt you 24/7, in order of negative impact on your daily life (I know you have more than 3, but let's work with 3 for now).
- Describe each of your 3 symptoms and how each one impacts your daily life, family, work, and any other situation.
- Describe how it would feel if your 3 most bothersome symptoms disappeared or

lessened to the point where they did not interfere with your daily life.

- What do you hope to get from reading and following the guidelines in this book?
- Set a calendar reminder for 6 months to revisit this letter and ask yourself the same questions as above. Compare your thoughts. How has your life changed in the past 6 months?

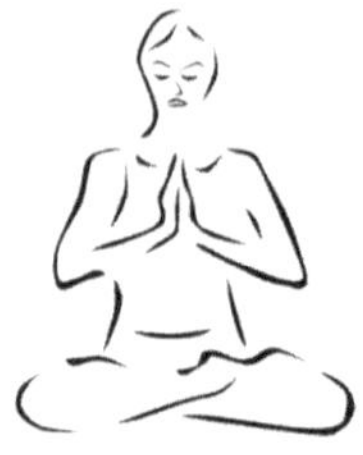

JOURNAL BREAK

A Time to *PAUSE* and Reflect

Name your 3 most bothersome symptoms, the ones that haunt you 24/7, in order of negative impact on your daily life (I know you have more than 3, but let's work with 3 for now).

____

____

____

____

____

____

Describe each of your 3 symptoms and how each one impacts your daily life, family, work, and any other situation.

Describe how it would feel if your 3 most bother-some symptoms disappeared or lessened to the point where they did not interfere with your daily life.

____

____

____

____

____

____

____

____

____

What do you hope to get from reading and following the guidelines in this book?

____

____

____

____

____

____

____

____

____

____

Set a calendar reminder for 6 months to revisit this letter and ask yourself the same questions as above. Compare your thoughts. How has your life changed in the past 6 months?

____

____

____

____

____

____

____

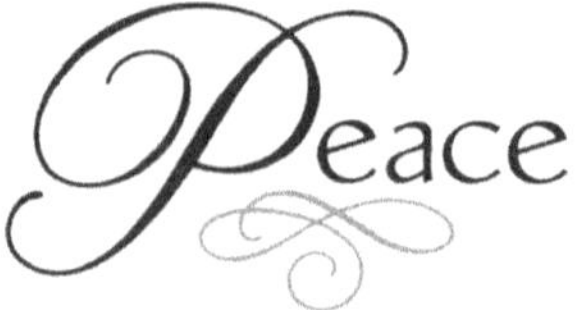

Chapter 2
WIN THE FIGHT AGAINST MENOPAUSE

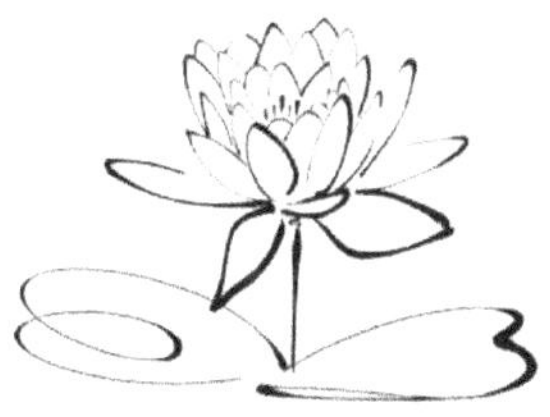

The Little Girl Inside Myself

There is a little girl who I see inside myself,
like the story in the novel sitting on the shelf.

The little girl becomes a woman, who is someone's wife,
and there begins the story, the story of my life.

It is a story of happiness, a story of pain,
a story of experience, experience to gain.

The story of my life is not an easy one to tell,
for it is a story like heaven, a story like hell.

I do not mean to frighten you,

I do not mean to scare,
I do not mean that my story is a total nightmare.

There are times of happiness, times of cheer,
there are times when my life to me is very dear.

For my life is one that was chosen to be,
I will be happy with what I have, even though it isn't me.

I cannot go on for the novel is too long,
I must put it back on the shelf,
and remember that I am strong.

~ Dr. Renata

Did you ever ride a roller coaster as a child? If so, think about what the experience was like for a moment. I just read an article in which a theme park recently conducted an interview with park visitors and asked them how it feels to ride a roller coaster. The answers they received were fascinating, but one in particular caught my attention.

Parkgoer Anthony Rout said this: "Waiting in the car as people get on gives you butterflies of anticipation as your heart begins to beat faster, your adrenaline causes your body [to] tense, and as the car pulls away the smile on your face is wide. Palms get sweaty as you chug up the climb, jolting and wondering if this was the best idea, then as the top appears you hold your breath, wait, moments pass in a heartbeat, then whoosh, your hair and face taking the full force of the wind as you try to hold on, holding back the screams for the first few dips, until suddenly you feel you can't hold it in. But you're not alone as the entire train are screaming as you bank the bend and dip, rush and find you are barely holding on, so you let go and allow your arms to wave in the air. The sudden clunk and slowing down is like a welcome friend, there to remind you that it's done, it's over, relax and get back in line."[1]

The change associated with menopause is almost like riding a roller coaster! When you are anticipating it, your heart begins to beat a little faster as you ponder middle age; your palms and face often get sweaty from the hot flashes; your emotions seem to fluctuate, making you feel out of control, and you often find yourself holding back screams because you're barely holding on. Once you learn to manage it, things slow down. You find out the ride is not that bad after all and possibly enjoyable. According to medical professionals on WebMD, here are some tips that might make it easier for you to handle those fluctuating emotions:

- Exercise and eat healthy.
- Find a self-calming skill to practice, such as yoga, meditation, or rhythmic breathing.
- Avoid alcohol.
- Engage in a creative outlet that fosters a sense of achievement.
- Stay connected with your family and community.
- Nurture your friendships.[2]

It's OK to embrace the change. Change, like any other life shift, may be frightening and unsettling. When it comes to menopause and perimenopause, talking about it isn't always easy— even considered taboo until recently. However, it's critical to be aware of what's going on in your body and approach the next chapter of your life with self-compassion.

When you venture into unfamiliar terrain, it's reassuring to know that many women have gone before you and come out stronger and wiser on the other side. You can win the fight against menopause!

We can beat the not-so-positive symptoms of menopause by adopting a healthy lifestyle that includes natural solutions. Every woman goes through menopause in her own way, so some natural remedies may help you feel better while others may not. Certain natural therapies can assist with more than one symptom of menopause, which may have an impact on your whole experience.

Activity: Committed to Winning the War

Winning the menopause war with your body and mind begins with winning daily mind and body battles. Some of us may experience numerous symptoms—maybe all forty at some point in our journeys—so it's important we get a handle on how to fight. First, let's get personal. I want you to focus on five of your most bothersome symptoms you are currently experiencing.

Use the following worksheet to:

1. List the top five (5) menopausal symptoms you are currently experiencing in order of severity.
2. Answer: How does each symptom negatively impact your daily life?
3. Set a realistic goal for change next to each symptom.
4. List a life-changing, positive outcome you might experience upon accomplishing your goal.

5 Battles & 5 Victories

Menopause Symptom (In order of severity)	How does this symptom affect your daily life?	What is your goal for change?	What is one positive outcome of meeting that goal?
1.			
2.			
3.			
4.			
5.			

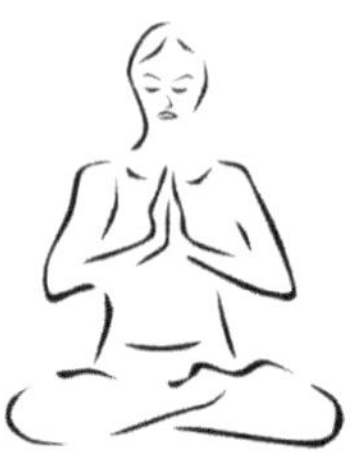

JOURNAL BREAK

A Time to *PAUSE* and Reflect

Take time to journal about how it would feel to win all the five battles you wrote out above?

____

____

____

____

____

____

____

____

____

____

____

____

____

____

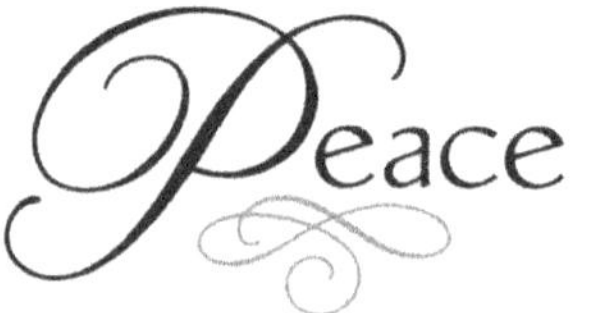

Peace

Chapter 3
THE MENOPAUSE MINDSET

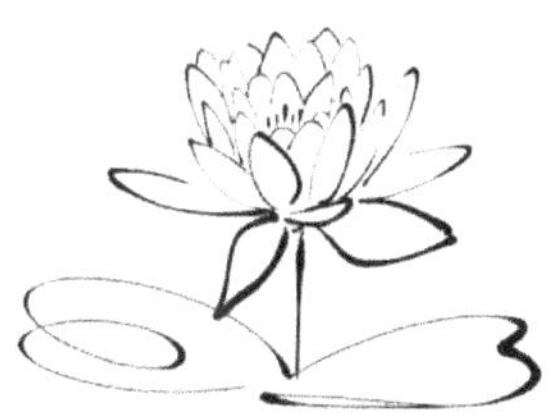

I Am Aware

I am a being that is aware of my emotions,
Yet not aware of all needed devotions.
My life to me is dear,
Yet there is daily hesitation and fear.
I want to be free to live my life as well as can be.
I want to be loved; I want to be me.

Myself is all I have,
That is all I need to be.
I take a breath,
I let it out,
I sing,
I shout.

I am a human,
I am free.
My future is a present to me.

~ Dr. Renata

Have you ever felt like you need to stop the clock ticking inside your mind and simply *be* in the present moment? That you just needed a break? Or better yet, a *pause*? To pause life for just a moment because you feel like you never have a moment to yourself?

As women, we tend to take the weight of a hundred responsibilities on our shoulders. So, in this chapter, I am going to help you get the "vacation" you've been needing. No, I am not booking you a flight to Hawaii or your favorite beach, but I am going to give you the secret to finding peace and tranquility in the midst of the roller-coaster ride that we call menopause . . . a *pause* for developing the right mindset.

The Meno*PAUSE* Mindset

Mindsets, according to research, play a crucial role in shaping life's results.[1] You can improve your health, reduce stress, and become more resilient to life's obstacles by understanding, adjusting, and altering your thinking. Mindsets are a collection of assumptions that let you reduce complicated worldviews into easily understandable bits of knowledge, which help us form opinions based on that information. For example, maybe you feel that going through menopause is the worst thing in the world or that following a diet would be difficult and depriving. These belief systems aid in the setting of your personal expectations, preparation for worst-case scenarios, and the making of decisions based on these assumptions. Simply put, what you think is going to shape the perception of what you experience. This is why is it so important to address our mindsets during menopause. And there's more . . .

Why Your Mindset Matters

Research shows that females are at a higher risk for developing mood disorders, including depression.[2] This has to do with a fluctuating hormone known as estrogen. The menopausal transition time is when estrogen levels become unstable, which often results in depression, anxiety, and other mood issues.

Your thoughts have the ability to influence your mood and the direction of your life, as well as impact certain experiences. Researchers have discovered that women who have a negative attitude toward menopause have more frequent and severe physical symptoms, whereas those who have a more favorable attitude toward menopause have fewer and milder symptoms.[3] This is groundbreaking!

Mood swings, irritability, anxiety, and sadness are all symptoms associated with low estrogen levels. Your moods can shift fast and furiously, taking you from laughing to sobbing in a matter of minutes. Have you ever experienced this?

The good news is *you* have the most control over your personal attitude, which greatly affects menopausal symptoms. Fortunately, optimism and resilience—the ability to adjust to life's challenges—are learned abilities that can be developed by everyone.[4, 5]

Winning the Estrogen Battle

Life is not fair, especially if you are a woman. As my mother always said, "Everything bad is for something good." I try to remember her words of wisdom, especially during the menopause roller-coaster battles. Each of us experiences a uniquely personal menopause journey, but it's often a battle we can win if we put our minds to it.

As I mentioned earlier, my menopause journey was a difficult and emotional one. Battling with my body and mind was a daily escapade. I am part of what is called the "sandwich generation," juggling the responsibilities of being a wife, mother, daughter, and caretaker to an ill father and brother, as well as caring for my elderly mom who had dementia. It all took a real toll on my mind and body. All of the symptoms you can find in the medical books about "menopause" were what I was experiencing.

I dreamed about getting my life back, not losing my mind, and feeling comfortable in my body once again. Through this, my mother was not able to give me advice because of her worsening dementia symptoms. During one of my darkest moments, I remembered her words of wisdom: "Everything bad is for something good." Those inspirational words from the woman I once knew as my role model made me strong in my weakest moments. I took a deep breath, looked in the mirror, and saw the woman I once was. With another deep breath, I promised myself to never allow the "*M* word" to distract me from living the life I deserved.

Later, I discovered the culprit: estrogen. What role does estrogen have on our moods? According to research, the hormone has mood-enhancing properties, implying that low levels might contribute to depression.

According to the SWAN study (Study of Women's Health Across the Nation), which was conducted over a ten-year period, as well as later studies, there is evidence suggesting that perimenopause is the start of an increased risk for depression in females. The studies suggest this may be because of psychosocial stress, the overall lifestyle, a lack of social support, sociodemographic characteristics, as well as a history of clinical depression. In general, there is strong evidence showing the hormonal changes that take place during the late reproductive years to postmenopausal years is a time of increased risk for depression in most women.[6, 7, 8]

Keeping my mother's wise words in the back of my mind, I wrote a note in my journal. "I am worthy and will not allow anything to stand in the way of the happiness I deserve." I took a deep breath and decided to allow this experience to make me stronger. Even though I was eating healthily, I adjusted my diet. I also stepped up my exercise routine and began swimming laps three or four times per week. I added a gentle ten-minute yoga and meditation practice each morning and at bedtime.

Then, my symptoms began to diminish. I felt closer to my old self again! However, thinking of the "*E* word" (estrogen, the culprit), I decided to get professional help. (I know I am a professional, but can a hairdresser cut their own hair? Maybe so, but how would it look?) I wanted faster results, even though I felt better than ever.

Though my gut told me not to—more of my mother's wise words: "Always listen to your gut" —I made an appointment with a naturopathic doctor who prescribed me BHRT, which stands for bioidentical hormone replacement therapy. BHRT is a natural alternative to synthetic HRT (hormone replacement therapy). BHRT reportedly does not cause serious side effects, so "Why not?" I thought. After my appointment, where I spent hundreds of dollars out-of-pocket since insurance does not cover this, I did some research and decided to give BHRT a try. For many women, BHRT is a lifesaver[9,10,11,], but it had the opposite effect on me.

After a few weeks, I looked in the mirror and, once again, did not recognize the face staring back at me. My face and body were changing—and not for the better! My clothes felt tighter. And when I stepped on the scale, I was fifteen pounds higher than before starting BHRT!

On top of my symptoms, I had an extra fifteen pounds to lose. I couldn't believe it! *What have I done?* I thought. I felt alone, afraid, and betrayed. After the tears fell, I actually screamed, blaming myself for not sticking to my plan, which had been working. I battled with my mind, asking, "How can I continue in my career if I cannot even help myself? What will my patients and peers think of me when they see the mess I have once again become?" My depressive symptoms returned.

After wallowing for a bit, I decided that ENOUGH was ENOUGH! I WOULD WIN the "M" battle! I intentionally chose a mindset instead of allowing my emotions to choose for me. Wow was it difficult to lose the weight I had gained while on BHRT, but with strength and perseverance, I won the "M" battle on my own by creating small goals for myself in the areas of food, yoga, and meditation and celebrating the victories along the way.

Like my journey, your menopause journey will require resilience, grit, and mental fortitude. I am not going to tell you it will be an easy fight, but I will tell you that it is possible to win. The only way you will not succeed is if you give up.

Angelica's Story

Angelica is an amazing woman who's navigated a lot throughout her life. She was my patient for many years. I remember the first day I met Angelica; she wore dark baggy clothes and was shy and depressed. She made such a transition with positive lifestyle changes that she became the subject of my research study. Angelica not only conquered her menopausal symptoms, but the change in her eating habits and lifestyle helped her prevent diabetes. She did not know much about menopause prior to experiencing it herself. She'd heard about some of the symptoms from her friends and family but never paid attention. In her experience, the "*M* word" ushered in a complete change to her body. "It's like you have no control with what you think and do."

Angelica was most surprised with the hot flashes. She felt "embarrassed" because this symptom, as she puts it, is "uncontrollable" and made her feel set apart in a group where others did not feel hot. Angelica, like many midlife women, wished someone had told her about menopause and the changes she might experience, the aches and pains and discomfort.

The bottom line is that Angelica, like all of the midlife women I interviewed, felt a negative impact on how she saw herself as a woman after the onset of her menopausal symptoms.

Angelica now refers to this stage in life as "passing to another level." When I asked Angelica if she believes the change with her nutrition and the addition of yoga and meditation to her routine changed who she was as a person, her reply was, "Yes, mentally I am more settled. I feel more at peace. It changed me totally!"

Remember, Angelica had never given much thought to menopause, even when she heard other women talking about it. Angelica brushed the dreaded "*M* word" aside and "moved on with her day." Her mother never experienced menopausal symptoms. Once, she asked her mother about menopause, and her mother said, "I don't know what that is." Angelica believes her mother was more confused about menopause than she was. Her younger sisters haven't gone through the "*M* stage" of their lives yet, so as she put it, "My support group was my gynecologist."

Angelica refers to her experience with menopause as *horrible*. Here are her words:

"It really affected my mood and health." She argued and fought with people, "even my own friends," she admitted. A turning point for her was when she realized the mood swings she struggled with were her own, and she couldn't blame others. "It was very emotional; I became depressed and developed anxiety. I'm doing much better now. I saw myself differently—I wasn't young anymore. It was as if I had reached a different level of life, especially because I could no longer have children.

"I can't say my symptoms were normal because to me, they weren't. I was in pain and uncomfortable for many months. After my last period, I had to go to a specialist because of the amount of bleeding I was experiencing. I was constantly changing my pads, more than when I had my period. There was also a sharp pain in my ovaries. I couldn't even move. The pain and bleeding lasted for months, making it difficult for me to do everything I wanted during that time. The pain wasn't only in my ovaries, but also the joints in my legs started to hurt. And I developed intense migraines.

"Menopause made losing weight more difficult for me. I ate less and exercised more but still did not lose weight. I tried many diets, such as the starch solution and the Mediterranean diet, but nothing worked for me. I used to be more active, staying out all night and still having energy during the day, but it's much harder in midlife. I try to stay active and go for walks when I can.

"One of the worst symptoms was hot flashes. It was embarrassing for me. Having a hot flash in front of people who are not sweating is strange, especially when they say things like, "It's cold" or "It's *not* hot!" while I'm fanning myself because I'm too hot. I went to a Christmas party with my daughter. I was wearing a pair of high boots. I looked so good that day, up until the hot flashes began. I felt as if everyone was staring at me. I was so embarrassed that I left the party early. The boots may have triggered the hot flashes, so I was nervous to wear them again. That wasn't the only time I experienced something like that, so now I go places prepared. I carry folding fans everywhere. People even gift them to me now, and I have collected some from other countries.

"Menopause also affected my sex life. Sex became painful and unenjoyable. This is when is started to feel like a chore, rather than something of pleasure. I felt as if I was doing it to please my partner, and that's not fair to either of us. If I'm going to have sex, I deserve to enjoy it.

"While the menopause transition was difficult for me, I feel more settled and at peace now. I have learned to feel comfortable in my body again. I can't go back in time, so all I can do now is accept who I am and continue to work on myself. When it comes to menopause, my advice for women is to learn how to deal with your symptoms and accept the fact your body isn't like it was before. I feel better than ever since I learned to accept myself and this new phase of my life. With healthy eating and practicing meditation and yoga on a regular basis, I have been feeling better than ever."[12]

The Secret PAUSE Formula

Take a *pause* from your menopause and learn how to use nutrition, yoga, and meditation to help with weight loss, bloating, and stress and get your life back!

1. **Nutrition:** Find foods from each food group that you can eat without gaining weight and feeling bloated.
2. **Yoga:** Learn to develop a personalized mini (light) yoga stretch routine to help decrease stress and control mood swings.
3. **Meditation:** Learn to use breathing techniques to calm your body and mind.

The *P.A.U.S.E.* Formula for Vibrancy, Health, and Happiness

Now, it's time for the vacation—I mean *pause*—that I promised you. In developing the mindset needed to feel like yourself again, you must remember these five words using the acronym *P.A.U.S.E.*

P: Positivity
A: Aspirations
U: Understanding
S: Self-care
E: Encouragement

Positivity: Always focus on the positive.

When bad things happen, how do you handle it? Is it easy to smile when your situation is less than ideal? It takes work to choose to remain happy through every situation. You can begin by recognizing the positive effects of menopause on you. Many women, for example, experience liberation with the ending of their monthly cycles.[13] Keep a daily gratitude diary in which you write down the things you are grateful for to develop a more positive view.

My biggest issue with the dreaded "*M* word" was weight gain, which was a problem for me even before menopause. I remember one time, in particular, looking in the mirror after squeezing my bigger body into my work clothes. I broke down and cried, then called out sick that day. I felt guilty, but I was sick . . . sick of my body!

After I spent hours sobbing in my bed and hiding under my covers, I thought about how it felt looking into that mirror and seeing a stranger staring at me. I promised myself to never feel like that again. Taking a deep breath, I said out loud, "Crying, hiding in bed, and calling out of work will not solve my problem." I had to get rid of the negative thoughts that were floating in my head. I had to think positively, no matter how I felt. So I walked over to my desk and grabbed a few sticky notes. I wrote several positive affirmations, one per note. I was so determined that by the end of that day, I had written 365 positive affirmations on 365 sticky notes. No, I did not stick them all on my mirror at once. I decided that each night, I would stick one positive affirmation note on the mirror. That minor task of putting a sticky note with a positive affirmation on my mirror every night when I brushed my teeth changed my mindset in the morning, allowing me to begin the day on a new road toward "*M* recovery."

Aspirations: Always have a goal to look forward to that will better your life.

Symptoms of menopause can be unpredictable.[14] It may seem as if your life and body are spinning out of control, so taking action to achieve a personal goal may be extremely motivating. This goal allows you to take back at least some control over your life. Small achievements may have a major influence on your health and wellbeing, so whether you choose to write a book, pick up a new hobby, start dating again, volunteer with a local organization, or join a support group, it all counts as progress.

Having aspirations or goals aids in the initiation of new behaviors, focuses the direction of our concentration, and furthers our momentum in life, which makes us feel productive as human beings.

Goals can also help us feel more in control of our lives, especially when menopause has you feeling out of control. Your life is not over just because your period is; you must find something to look forward to that inspires you to keep moving forward.

With that, let's take some time to answer these questions, and we'll get back to the acronym *P.A.U.S.E.* in a moment:

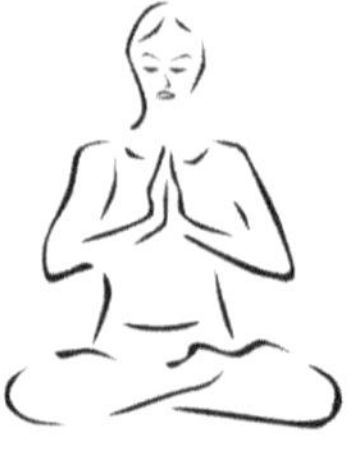

JOURNAL BREAK

A Time to *PAUSE* and Reflect

Take a moment to read and think about the following questions:

- What are your 3 main health goals?
- Are you tracking the above 3 goals?
- Where do you see yourself in your "perfect" near future?
- In 1 year?
- In 5 years?
- What do you hope to get out of reading this book?
- What is something that currently upsets you in life?
- Name at least one positive in that situation.
- What are you most grateful for in life?

Now, use the following 3 pages to journal your thoughts to those questions.

What are your 3 main health goals?

1. _______________________________________
2. _______________________________________
3. _______________________________________

Are you tracking those 3 goals? If so, how and does the tracking help you progress toward them? If you're not already tracking them, how might you start?

____

____

____

____

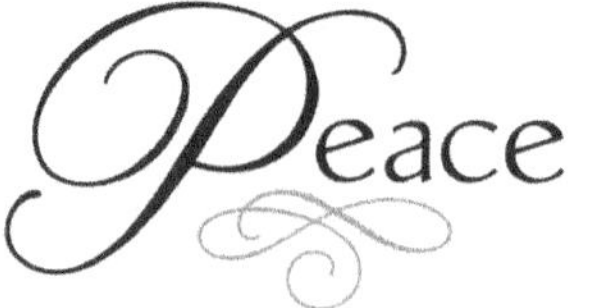

Where do you see yourself in your "perfect" near future (3 to 6 months out)?

____

____

____

____

In 1 year?

____

____

____

____

In 5 years?

____

____

____

____

____

What do you hope to get out of reading this book?

____

____

____

____

What is something that upsets you in life?

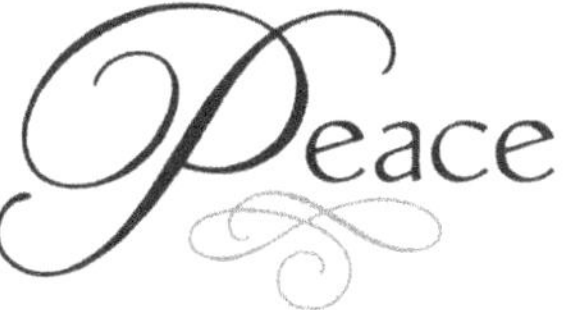

Name at least one positive in that situation?

____

____

____

____

What are you most grateful for in life?

____

____

____

____

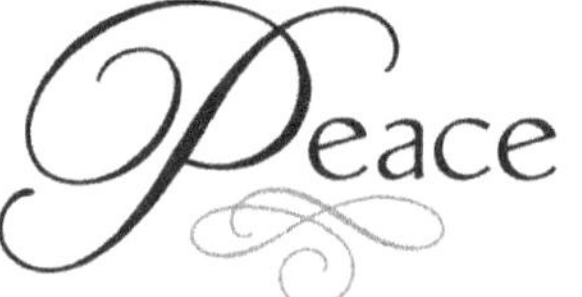

You can't manage what you don't measure, and you can't improve what you don't manage correctly. Therefore, knowing who you are and setting goals can assist you in accomplishing all these things and more. Now, let's move on with the P.A.U.S.E. acronym for developing a mindset and strategies that will help you on your "*M* journey."

Understanding: Understand your symptoms and be sure to get checked and cleared by a medical doctor.[15]

Being in tune with our midlife bodies is key to finding our best selves. It is especially important to keep up with medical appointments in midlife. Before beginning any self-care journey, make sure you are up to date with all of your medical visits and assessments. Seeking therapeutic assistance for menopausal symptoms has to do with quality of life.

Please note: It is imperative you consult a specialist in the event you experience vaginal bleeding after menopause. Don't be afraid to express this or any other concern with your medical doctor. During midlife, your doctor will likely advise you to have preventive screening procedures, such as colonoscopies and mammography. Once you are medically cleared, your symptoms are more likely to be related to the menopausal transition rather than a serious medical condition. Remember, all of our "*M* journeys" are unique, so don't compare yours to others.

If you are current with medical exams and do not have unusual symptoms needing medical attention, such as vaginal bleeding and abdominal pain, and have been told by your medical doctor that your symptoms are due to menopause, then my *P.A.U.S.E.* formula will pause your most bothersome symptoms.

I've included a quick checklist so you can be sure you're ready to move forward with the formula.

Ask yourself the following ten (10) questions and use the chart below to mark your answers.

QUESTION	YES	NO
1. Have I been checked and cleared by a medical doctor?		
2. Has my doctor confirmed that my symptoms are due to menopause?		
3. Have I been experiencing mood swings?		
4. Am I more emotional lately?		
5. Am I experiencing brain fog?		
6. Do I feel more tired than usual?		
7. Do I have a harder time falling and staying asleep?		
8. Do I get bloated after meals?		
9. Do I gain weight easier than before?		
10. Am I ready to get my life back?		

*If you answered *yes* to question #1 and *yes* to one or more of questions #2–10, then you can move on and benefit from this book.

Some common symptoms of menopause, though minor, disrupt midlife women's lives and become debilitating. Some menopausal symptoms are so debilitating that our ability to maintain relationships or even function on a daily basis becomes almost impossible. Many midlife women ignore their symptoms and believe they are losing their minds when, in fact, all of this has to do with hormone loss and aging. As a midlife woman, you deserve health, happiness, and a high quality of life.

Self-Care: The S in Our *P.A.U.S.E.* Acronym

Healthy eating habits, being physically active, de-stressing, listening to your body, and taking a *pause* when needed are all part of self-care.[16] It's important to do things that make you happy and enjoy life at any age. When was the last time you did something nice for *you*? Pause and think about this and use the space below to write down your thoughts.

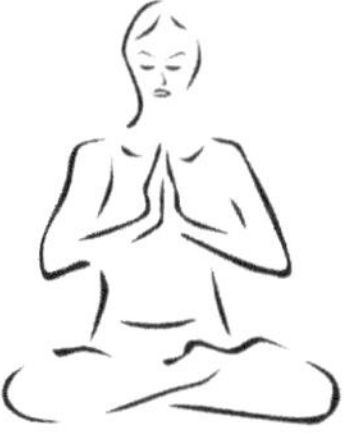

JOURNAL BREAK

A Time to *PAUSE* and Reflect

What have you done for *you* lately in terms of Self-Care?

____

____

____

____

____

____

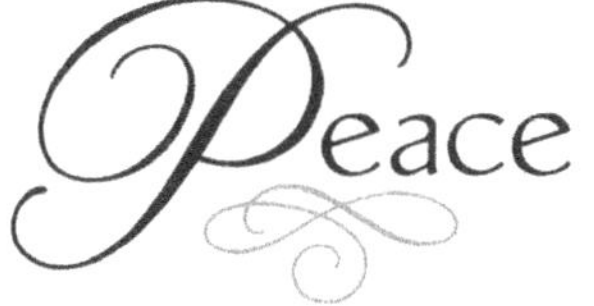

As women and mothers, we naturally care for others.[17] We want to make sure that everyone around us has everything they need while, at times, forgetting about what we need. You are important too, and if you do not take care of yourself, you will not be in a position to help others.

I was the youngest in my family and known as the caretaker. Yes, the youngest and the caretaker; you read that correctly. I was born in the Czech Republic, and at the age of four, escaped with my parents and brother to Austria. We lived there for nine months, then set out for America. When we arrived in the USA, I was still young, and I absorbed English faster than my brother and parents. This made me the official family translator. My brother was fifteen years old, and my parents were both forty-four years old when I was born. I became used to looking out for my small family. It kept me busy and became a way of life. Though my family never asked me to care for them, it was a natural thing for me to do. This arrangement took its toll on me when my father was diagnosed with stomach cancer. I was only twenty-six. I had a young family of my own, yet I also became the caretaker for my ailing father—until the end.

After my father passed away, my brother had a stroke, and his ex-wife left him in the hospital with the clothes on his back. I took him in and nursed him back to health.

A few years later, my mother, who was my best friend, developed dementia, which lasted for nine long years. My family and I cared for her in our home until she had to be transported into hospice care. Being busy caring for others 24/7 and not having much (if any) down time was not healthy physically or mentally. My lack of self-care got so out of hand that when my husband lost his job, I took on two side jobs in addition to my full-time job. Working three jobs seven days a week became the norm. This continued until one day, a patient told me that I deserved a vacation. Those words hit me just right.

I had been commuting two to three hours each way via car, train, and two subways, sweating in the summer (and bringing extra clothes and drying my hair in the bathroom because midlife does that!) and freezing in the winter (though sweating under my coat). I will never forget one particular day I wanted to call out sick. I wasn't feeling well, but my robotic brain put self-care last on my to-do list. That morning, while on the railroad, I was in a horrific train accident. The train crashed into the wall at the station. I was crushed by a large male, who was thrown on top of me. When I got the strength to stand up, all I could think about was, "I have to get to work!" As I limped to the subway station, I was stopped by a news team. To this day, I have tangible, video proof of my lack of self-care.

I am embarrassed to watch the clip (which can still be found on YouTube). On the national news, after experiencing the trauma of this accident, I said, "I have to get to work." I then showed the news team my bruised arm. I managed to get to work somehow—and only ten minutes late! As I hobbled past the staff to my office, I even apologized that I was late! Well, that was a *big* wake up call. I needed a *PAUSE*! Two hours later, my head began to spin, and I couldn't stand up straight. It turned out, my blood pressure was elevated, and I had a Grade Two concussion. I also suffered nerve damage to the right side of my body and a bruised shoulder, arm, and leg.

It was the moments when my head was spinning that thoughts of dying crossed my mind, and I realized that self-care is not a privilege; it is a necessity. I used my time off to recover, but my stubborn self did one more thing indicative of my old habits; I accepted an offer to create and teach a master level class at the city university. Teaching at that higher level had been on my bucket list, so how could I turn it down? Once again, instead of resting, I designed the curriculum and drove twenty miles to the school, all against my doctors' orders.

My lack of self-care put me on bedrest for an extra two weeks and taught me a big lesson. I decided to take fifteen minutes to do light yoga and meditation upon waking and before going to bed. Just that minor addition to my daily routine changed my life.

That was years ago. Since then, I always take a *PAUSE* and plan self-care times and days, allowing myself to recharge and care for others by caring for myself. I learned the importance of self-care the hard way. I hope you should learn it simply by trusting me because you are worth it.

Self-care can take various forms, and it is unique to everyone. You must allow yourself to accept your body, mind, and emotions so you can acknowledge when you need to take time to refuel.

Imagine driving your car until you run out of gas and then trying to drive further. What would happen? Nothing! Neither you nor your car would go anywhere because you wouldn't have enough gas or fuel to make it to another destination. Our bodies operate the same way. We have an "fuel gauge" that lets us know when it is time to fill back up. The problem is that, many times, we ignore the signals of fatigue or irritability and push ourselves until we cannot go any further. Just as we intentionally go the gas station and fill up our cars, we must intentionally do something nice for ourselves. Sometimes, it's saying no when our schedule is full, then not feeling bad about it. Other times, it is taking time to unwind with a warm bath or indulging in your favorite snack. Whatever relaxes you, find time to do it.

Activity: Have Fun!

What is your favorite activity that brings you the greatest joy? Use the rest of this page to write your thoughts on which activities you enjoy. (Make time for at least one this week!)

____

____

____

____

____

____

____

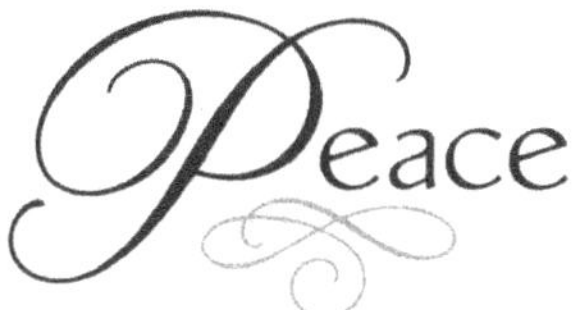

Encouragement: Encourage yourself and others.

When going through menopause, it is important to find "your people"—a group of relatable women. The times I was alone in my menopause battle were the hardest. Trying to motivate myself when I felt like no one understood what I was going through was tough. There were times along my journey when I felt like I had a lot of support and times when I felt completely alone. It was when I connected with other midlife women experiencing similar symptoms that I could stay on track and win the menopause battle.

The Happiness Jar

I've always been drawn to psychology books and health food stores. When I was twelve, my mother allowed me to walk to the store by myself. That first "grown up" outing is etched into my memory. I was so excited and felt so grown up.

One day, I walked three miles to the bookstore and bought a wellness book with my babysitting money. I was thrilled to soak in the wealth of information I found inside that book. It was about the importance of nutrition and physical activity.

There was even a chapter on yoga and meditation. As an immigrant child from a meat and potatoes country, much of the information was new to me. Carrying my newfound love, I ran across the street as excitement roared in my mind and body. Looking up, I read the sign: "Health Food Store." I had seen the sign on many occasions. In fact, the supermarket my parents shopped in was right next door. I bought a few items with the last of my babysitting money I had grabbed from my "happiness jar." As I left the store, I spotted a box with the word "FREE" written on it. Inside was a cookbook titled *Laurel's Kitchen*. I grabbed the cookbook with my free hand, held the wellness book and other items I purchased with the other, and ran all the way home with the ingredients of what would become my career.

The happiness jar I created for my patients does not contain money. It is a jar filled with positive affirmations for women in my support groups. Each week, every group member receives an affirmation, which they use as inspiration to help achieve their weekly goals. The affirmations in the happiness jar are powerful, mind-changing tools. Sisters Norma and Diana, who are experiencing midlife together, have prevailed in even the toughest of times using affirmations to cope with their daily lives. In fact, Norma has created her own line of positive affirmation signs and stickers, which she gives to women in need.

During my twenty-plus-year career, I have led weekly wellness support groups, which are a vital part of the healing process. Support groups offer midlife women like us a positive environment, encouragement, and unity. Midlife women who join support groups find their people. I would love for you to join my Facebook groups and find your people and get access to free educational materials and support for your menopause journey.

Sometimes, we wait for others to acknowledge us or uplift us when we are down, and that does not always happen. This can make us feel disgruntled, especially if our hormones are all over the place. Therefore, it is imperative we learn how to encourage ourselves. While not always easy, it is possible. Here are a few tips to help you cheer yourself up when necessary:

- Focus on what is going right and not on what is going wrong.
- Celebrate the little wins. You may not have the results you want yet, but you can

take a moment right now to acknowledge any amount of progress you have accomplished so far.

- Have confidence that everything will work out in your favor.
- Use positive affirmations to help shape your thoughts.

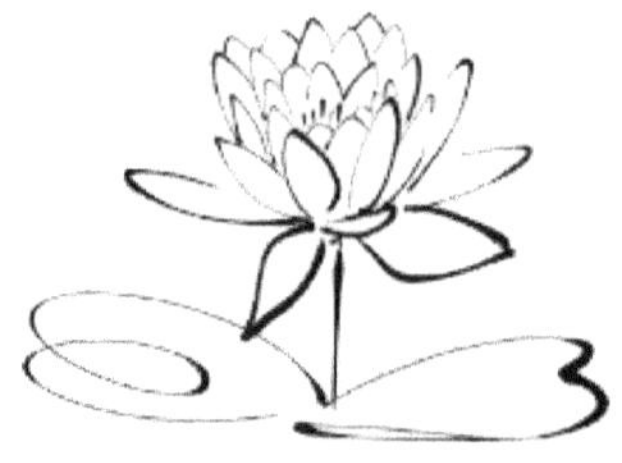

Let It Go

Let go of negativity and anxiety . . . Let it go.
Let go of muddled beliefs . . . of hesitation,
Misplaced thoughts or verses . . . Let them go.
Let go of wrong reason . . . Let it go.
Let go of dread and conclusions . . .
Let go of anticipation . . .
Just let them go.

Don't check the elements, don't investigate. Let it go.
Don't say a word, no one will acknowledge or notice . . .
Like foliage tumbling from a tree . . . Let it go.
Don't promise, broadcast . . . Let it go.
It wasn't worth it; it wasn't wanted . . .
It was what it was, and is just that . . .
place a grin on your façade,
and forevermore,
JUST LET IT GO!

~ Dr. Renata

My "go to" positive affirmation is one I shared with you earlier in this chapter—my mother's wise words: "Everything bad is for something good." Repeating these simple words every morning and before bed has changed my life and lifted me out of my darkest moments.

A student of mine was so inspired by these words that she had a plaque made for me. I keep the plaque on my desk and share these words with my patients. My mother's words of encouragement have helped countless women get through the toughest of times. I encourage you to write a few words that inspire *you*; create your own affirmation. If you want to use my mother's wise words of wisdom, we'd be honored. Repeat your affirmation often to allow for the healing of your mind and the release of negative thoughts. Here are some examples to get you started:

- "I am in the right place at the right time, doing the right thing." (Louise Hay)
- "The chance to love and be loved exists no matter where you are." (Oprah)
- "Am I good enough? Yes, I am." (Michelle Obama)

- "Nothing can dim the light that shines from within." (Maya Angelou)
- "Just for today, do not worry." (Dr. Mikao Usui)
- "I am successful. I am confident. I am powerful. I am strong. I am a woman." (Dr. Renata)

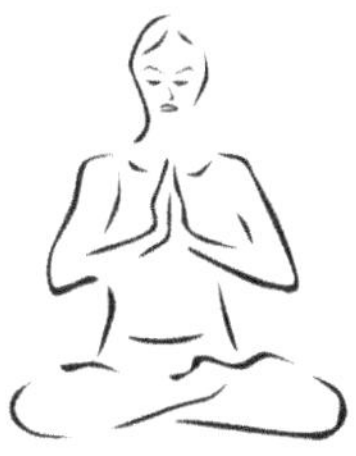

JOURNAL BREAK

A Time to *PAUSE* and Reflect

Activity: Write three to five affirmations that you will repeat daily and whenever you feel like life has knocked you down.

____

____

____

____

____

____

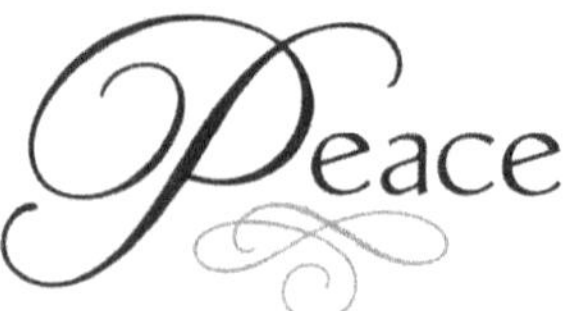

Peace

Chapter 4
YOU ARE NOT ALONE

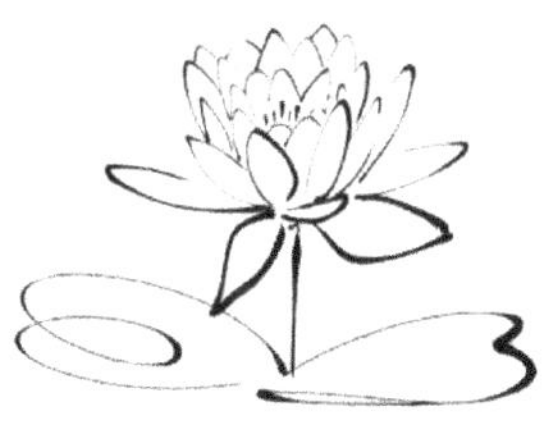

The Lonely One

Staring in the mirror,
Gazing at my face,
Why am I in this lonely place?

Can anybody hear me,
Is anybody here?
I'm crying deep inside, screaming from the fear.

~ Dr. Renata

I am delighted that more and more women are openly discussing menopause. Women used to suffer in silence, believing all of the unpleasant symptoms were "normal."[1] Well, while the symptoms are common, they do not have to be a part of your normal, everyday life.

As I previously stated, I've had the privilege of coaching and assisting many women who were seeking ways to manage menopause so it would no longer manage them. The one consistent piece, with the thousands of women I've had the honor of serving over the past twenty years, is they were overjoyed to learn they weren't alone. Here are a few stories from women just like you who learned to *pause* the symptoms of menopause.

Jenny: Night Sweats

"My most bothersome menopausal symptom was waking up during the night soaking wet from profuse sweating. I decreased the frequency and intensity of my intense night sweats through adding a weekly exercise routine and making intentional decisions with my beverages. I took Dr. Renata's advice and began wearing thin, loose-fitting pajamas to bed rather than warm fuzzy ones. I layered my outdoor clothing as well. This enabled me to take off layers as I needed, preventing excessive sweating and embarrassing moments. I found lowering the temperature in my bedroom to a little below comfortable helped keep my night sweats to a minimum. Another trick Dr. Renata taught me was to avoid spicy foods and caffeinated beverages and definitely stay away from alcohol. The most important thing I have done to help control those annoying and uncomfortable night sweats is to not stress about everything. This was a difficult thing to do since I have a "Type-A" personality. Through Dr. Renata's guidance, I lowered my stress level through simple meditation and yoga routines, which I practice when I wake up, before bed, and anytime stress rears its ugly head at me."

Patresse: Weight Gain

"I have worked at losing weight since gaining extra pounds during menopause. I changed how much I ate and what I ate and started walking often. I learned about nutrition and adapting a healthy lifestyle from Dr. Renata. I learned that I had to eat smaller portions to get the menopause weight off. Before I met Dr. Renata, I was eating late at night. Menopause had me up three to four times per night to use the bathroom. Instead of just going to the bathroom, I went to the kitchen to get a snack. Since I went through menopause early in life, I experienced symptoms for many years. I believe going through menopause has made me a better person. I feel stronger and more aware of my body and the changes women go through. I learned to accept menopause and my body. Keeping myself fit is very important at this stage in life. I continue with the activities I did before menopause, and I added walking home from work to burn extra calories. Walking has helped me stay active and manager my anxiety, and it has helped distract me from the other symptoms caused by menopause. Life changes as the years go by, but because of my experience with menopause, I feel more prepared for anything."

Diana: Mood Swings

"The most drastic change for me during menopause was the emotional shifts I experienced. I never thought I would go through that or that I could be so emotional and sensitive. I was never that way growing up. Suddenly, I was fine one minute, but then a leaf fell off of a tree, and I would just start crying. I was also surprised with how tired I was all of the time. But if there was one menopausal symptom that I could get rid of, it would definitely be the emotional "yoyo." I can handle everything else, but the up-and-down emotional swings and crying like a baby out of nowhere—that can go!

I remind myself to stay positive and think positive thoughts. When I need someone to talk to someone, I always call my sister. It works every time because she makes me laugh. It is important to be surrounded by loved ones. Dr. Renata has taught me that practicing self-care, including adapting to a healthy diet (nutrition) and lifestyle changes make the whole difference when it comes to mood swings. The bottom line is that you can't go through this alone. This truth helped me get through some tough times in my worst menopausal years. I learned how to cope with things and how not to stay in a cloud of depression. My mom taught me that our bodies go through many different changes and to love myself just the way I am. My entire family was a great support system for me during menopause."

The Power of Connection

Today, we are more "connected" than ever before.[2] You name it—Instagram, Facebook, Tik-Tok, LinkedIn, Snapchat, and so on—we have access to people through a small device that fits into the palms of our hands. However, are we really *connected?* There is a big difference between getting a "like" or "comment" on a social media post and getting real-time, live feedback from a friend during a phone call or making eye contact with someone who likes us. This same principle applies to our menopause journey. Connecting with like-minded women and sharing our stories gives us a safe space to overcome our struggles and help others overcome theirs. We need a sense of community to feel supported and also learn from others.[3]

My community of midlife women is an important group of like-minded individuals. The cohesiveness stems from sharing our relatable situations, usually happening at similar times. Women coming together is a powerful team of individuals that can help one another through the toughest of times. We are always there for each other, no matter what life brings our way—whether it is a dreadful symptom suddenly taking over our lives or a positive situation we want to share and celebrate. We cry and laugh on each other's shoulders.

"Sharing these moments make us as one." Those words came straight one of women in our group. I am not only their leader but a peer as well. I understand their situations, no matter their backgrounds or differences. My group meets on a weekly basis and come from all walks of life, even from all over the globe. Those who live near each other have met in person and have become buddies who walk and talk and are growing old together. Virtual connections have made our group even stronger than I ever thought possible. We are able to comfort each other day and night. Whenever we need a shoulder to cry on or a laugh or smile to share, someone is always there.

We have an online support group and a "24/7" texting system for sharing anything at any given moment. I am always available, so group members can text me if they are feeling upset, happy, or just want to say hello. They also have access to my Facebook groups, including a wellness nutrition group and a yoga and meditation group. Patients can also listen to my weekly podcasts and set up one-on-one sessions with me—I am there for them. I love my community of like-minded midlife women, and they love my program!

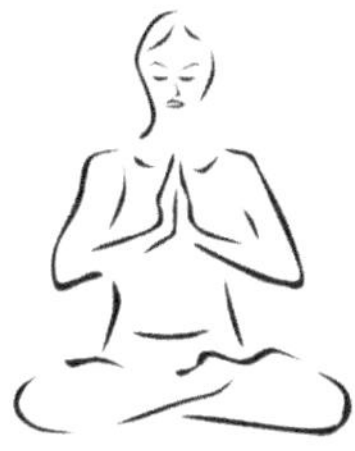

JOURNAL BREAK

A Time to *PAUSE* and Reflect

Activity: Share Your Story

This week, share your story with someone who might benefit from it. Then write about your experience and what *you* learned about sharing.

____

____

____

____

____

____

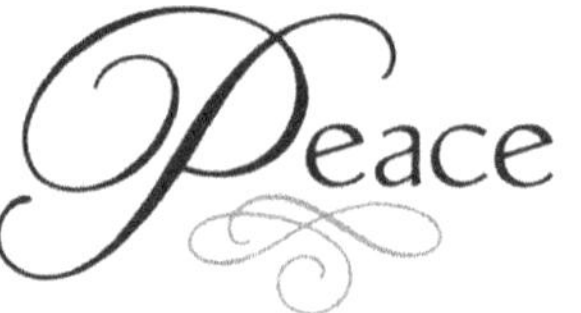

Chapter 5
WHAT YOU EAT MATTERS

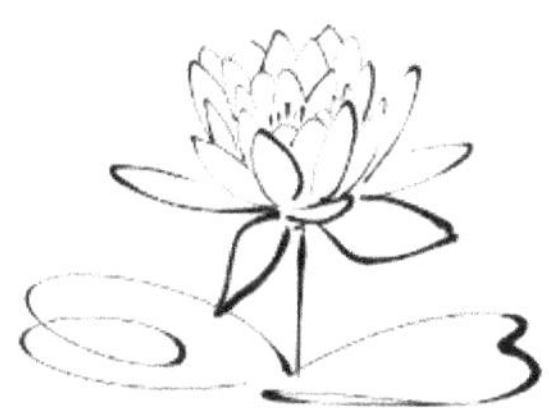

Have you ever heard the expression, "You are what you eat"? This simply means, what you put in your body determines whether you are healthy or not. Some of the risk factors and symptoms associated with aging and menopause are unavoidable. However, healthy eating can help avoid or alleviate some of the symptoms that can arise during and after menopause. In this chapter, I talk about *why* it's important to have a healthy diet and what you should eat for maximum relief from symptoms.[1]

Why Eating Matters in Menopause

Healthy eating is a crucial aspect of self-care throughout menopause. It provides your body with essential minerals like calcium and vitamin D. It assists in maintaining a healthy weight. It can also lower your risk of health concerns associated with menopause, such as heart disease and osteoporosis.[2]

The Keys to a Feel-Good Menopausal Food Plan

There are several key items to include in your food plan, which will help alleviate menopausal symptoms while allowing for necessary nutrients so we age gracefully and healthfully. These key foods include whole foods, fresh fruits and vegetables, 100 percent whole grains, high-quality dairy—such as Greek yogurt—and foods rich in phytoestrogens and healthy fats, such as Omega-3.[3]

Consume Foods Rich in:

- Plant estrogens, otherwise known as phytoestrogens
- Fresh organic non-starchy vegetables and fruits (limit fruit to 1–2 servings per day)
- Calcium, magnesium, and vitamin D
- Low-fat organic Greek yogurt, raw organic nuts and seeds

- Omega-3 fatty acids
- Wild-caught salmon and other fatty fish, raw organic nuts, and organic ground flax seeds

Assignment: Your Food and Mood Diary

Track what you eat, your symptoms, and your mood (and swings) for one week, and let's find the foods that may be the culprits triggering you mentally and emotionally. Knowing which foods trigger your mood can help you to take control of this symptom, helping you feel better mentally and physically.

Use the Daily Food/Mood tracking pages below to record all of the food items and beverages you ingest for the next three days. Keeping track of your daily food intake will help you to identify food and mood triggers and help get you back to feeling more emotionally stable.

Food/Mood Diary Instructions

The best way to track your foods and moods is to write as you eat or pre-plan your daily meals and snacks the night before. Filling out your Food/Mood sheets from memory is not an accurate method, and you will not reap the benefits of knowing your true food triggers.

DAILY FOOD/MOOD LOG

DAY 1

Name: ____

Date: ____

Water: 8 (8-oz glasses):
[ ] [ ] [ ] [ ] [ ] [ ] [ ] [ ]
Steps Taken: ____________________
Exercise (Type and Minutes):

____

Write the foods you eat and the beverages you drink for 3 days and note what your mood is like before/after your meals/snacks, be as specific as you can. Make note of your physical activity and water intake as well.

Time	Meal#1	Mood
		☹ ☹ 😐 🙂 😊
Time	Snack #1 (Optional)	Mood
		☹ ☹ 😐 🙂 😊
Time	Meal #2	Mood
		☹ ☹ 😐 🙂 😊
Time	Snack #2 (Optional)	Mood
		☹ ☹ 😐 🙂 😊
Time	Meal #3	Mood
		☹ ☹ 😐 🙂 😊
Time	Snack #3 (Optional)	Mood
		☹ ☹ 😐 🙂 😊

DAY 2

Name: ___________________________________

Date: ___________________________________

Water: 8 (8-oz glasses):
[ ] [ ] [ ] [ ] [ ] [ ] [ ] [ ]
Steps Taken: _______________________
Exercise (Type and Minutes):

____

Write the foods you eat and the beverages you drink for 3 days and note what your mood is like before/after your meals/snacks, be as specific as you can. Make note of your physical activity and water intake as well.

Time	Meal#1	Mood 😞 🙁 😐 🙂 😊
Time	Snack #1 (Optional)	Mood 😞 🙁 😐 🙂 😊
Time	Meal #2	Mood 😞 🙁 😐 🙂 😊
Time	Snack #2 (Optional)	Mood 😞 🙁 😐 🙂 😊
Time	Meal #3	Mood 😞 🙁 😐 🙂 😊
Time	Snack #3 (Optional)	Mood 😞 🙁 😐 🙂 😊

DAY 3

Name: _______________________________________

Date: _______________________________________

Water: 8 (8-oz glasses):
[ ] [ ] [ ] [ ] [ ] [ ] [ ] [ ]
Steps Taken: _______________________
Exercise (Type and Minutes):

____

Write the foods you eat and the beverages you drink for 3 days and note what your mood is like before/after your meals/snacks, be as specific as you can. Make note of your physical activity and water intake as well.

Time	Meal#1	Mood
Time	Snack #1 (Optional)	Mood
Time	Meal #2	Mood
Time	Snack #2 (Optional)	Mood
Time	Meal #3	Mood
Time	Snack #3 (Optional)	Mood

Chapter 6
HEALTHY EATING CASE STUDIES

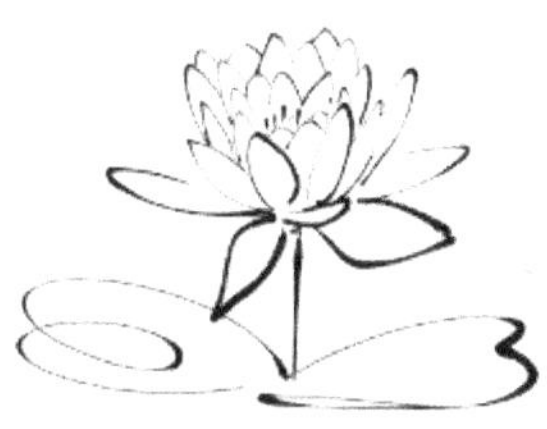

Lisa, one of the sixteen women interviewed for this book, began gaining weight rapidly during the beginning of her menopausal transition. Every time she stepped on her scale the number rose higher. She said it had gotten so out-of-control that she could not button her pants, which once fit loosely on her. Lisa was even more devastated when she was in the dressing room at her local department store, and nothing fit. To her disbelief, she had gone up two dress sizes. This caused Lisa's mood to change from a happy-go-lucky woman to a sad, depressed, and reclusive one. Lisa once said, "I hide in bed most weekends, wishing I could go out like I used to." Lisa like most of the other women, described her mood swings and depression as "unbearable."

Lisa was so desperate to lose the weight she had gained, she bought over-the-counter weight-loss pills that caused heart palpitations, which sent her to the emergency room. The blood tests showed Lisa's thyroid levels were slightly low. The doctor suggested she take a low-dose medicine (Synthroid), which would most likely help her lose weight. Well, not only did Lisa *not* lose weight, but one month later, she had added another ten pounds on to her already overweight body. This is when she found me through a Google search.

I helped Lisa make changes to her eating habits, and within a few weeks, she watched the number on the scale go down. With her new eating habits and lifestyle changes, Lisa lost the weight she had gained and felt better mentally than she did in her earlier years.

Like Lisa, Angelica also experienced drastic mood changes along with weight gain when her menopausal journey began. In fact, Angelica told me that she not only gained twenty pounds in the first month of her transitional journey, but she was so bloated, her stomach looked bigger than when she was pregnant. Unlike Lisa, Angelica also experienced "extreme" hot flashes. She described them as "coming out of nowhere." Angelica's hot flashes had gotten so out-of-control that she stopped socializing altogether. Like a vicious cycle, her hermit-like sedentary lifestyle led to depression and anxiety and even more weight gain.

Angelica was desperate to lose the weight she had gained. Depressed and upset that she let herself get to the point of tipping the scale at 205 pounds, Angelica knew she had to make a change. Crying during her first session with me, Angelica vowed to never feel that way again. My first piece of advice was to focus on little goals to achieve her ultimate goal.

Before our meeting, both Lisa and Angelica felt helpless, having tried every fad diet and numerous concoctions to help them lose weight. Nothing worked. After both women eliminated the foods that were the culprits of their symptoms, added healthy food choices to their daily diets, adapted a healthier lifestyle through practicing light yoga three to four times each week, and adding a short meditation routine upon waking and at bedtime, they were stunned with the changes they experienced.

On the first day, they both reported feeling "much better" and having more energy. Within two weeks, Lisa lost four pounds, and Angelica lost five pounds. The weight they had gained melted off, and both reported they felt "alive again." Within six months, both women reached their ideal body weight and felt relief, even "amazing."

It was those raw moments of truth that Lisa and Angelica realized the only way they would fail and never achieve their goals was to give up. Both women overcame the emotional menopausal roller coaster of weight gain and are now living their lives to the fullest capacity. Lisa and Angelica agree that if they hadn't made the changes they made, they would have not been able to enjoy the best golden years of their lives.

Common Causes of Menopausal Weight Gain

The probable cause for Lisa and Angelica's weight gain during their transition was the decline in their estrogen levels. Estrogens are essential in the body and contribute to different bodily functions related to cardiovascular health and bone health and help regulate metabolic status. The transition into menopause is often accompanied by a decrease in metabolic rate, which lowers the rate the body efficiently burns calories. An increase in fatty tissue (adiposity) occurs, mainly in the middle part of the body. These changes in estrogen levels during the menopausal phase leads to weight gain and a higher body mass index, which increases the risk of obesity, diabetes, and other health related risk factors.[1,2]

The good news is there are natural ways to help alleviate the symptoms associated with lower estrogen levels, namely weight gain. The main method is through specific food choices.

Chapter 7
RECIPES FOR RELIEF

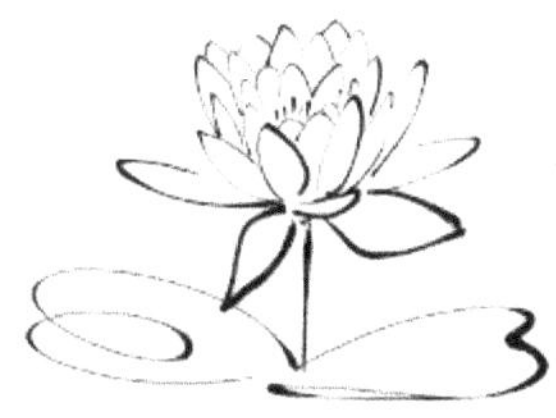

Now that you've learned why eating a nutritious diet is so important and read a couple of case studies, hopefully you know that since healthy food choices worked for Lisa and Angelica, they could work for you too. I am not saying food choice is the magic, cure-all pill, but I am saying that it will help you in the long run.

Therefore, it's time to begin cooking! In this chapter, I share a few tried-and-true dishes that will help you receive the nourishment you need while also pleasing your palate. As with any new program or diet, please consult with your doctor first.

Most menopausal women find relief for symptoms through adding certain foods to their daily diet. Below are four of the most common symptoms the women I interviewed suffered with and a food cure you, like my patients, might find relief by trying.

1. Menopause Symptom: Weight Gain

Food Cure = Avocados

Avocados are green pear-shaped fruits known for their rich monounsaturated fats and oleic fatty acids, which have been shown to have anti-inflammatory effects. Little did we know there is more to avocados than just being a good source of fat! Avocados are highly nutritious as good sources of vitamins C, E, and K.[1] They are also high in potassium and rich in fiber, which studies show help promote feeling fuller longer and aid in the management of healthy weights. A study that observed the nutritional patterns of Americans showed that people who consumed avocados tended to eat a more nutrient-rich diet, had lower metabolic syndrome, and had lower body weight than those who did not.[2] This study also showed how those who ate avocados had lower body mass indices and smaller waist circumferences.[3] Consuming avocados daily is encouraged to help with satiety, promote a healthy weight loss, and support metabolic health.

2. Menopausal Symptoms: Mood Swings, Anxiety

Food Cure = Turmeric and black pepper

During the menopausal transition in life, women experience hormone fluctuations and physical changes leading to emotional imbalances, which lead to mood swings. Studies show that 23 percent of women experience mood disorder symptoms during the menopausal transition.[4]

Turmeric is a traditional Indian spice historically used in ayurvedic medicine and is part of the ginger family. Curcumin is a major component of turmeric that has gained a lot of interest for its powerful health benefits, which include aiding in the management of inflammatory conditions, metabolic syndrome, and anxiety, to name a few. Studies show that the main property of turmeric, curcumin, has potential anti-anxiety effects and is beneficial for mental health. This is possibly because of increasing serotonin and dopamine levels.[5] The health benefits of turmeric can be attributed to its antioxidant and anti-inflammatory effects, however, because of curcumin's poor bioavailability, turmeric should not be consumed alone. It is recommended that turmeric be combined with piperine, a compound found in black pepper, which has been shown to increase the absorption of turmeric by 2000 percent.[6]

I begin each day with a meditation and a soothing turmeric lemon detox tea. Adding turmeric and freshly squeezed lemon to filtered water gives me more energy than a cup of coffee. The anti-inflammatory properties in my homemade detox tea also help keep my mood stable throughout the day.

3. Menopause Symptom: Hot Flashes

Food Cure = Apples/Apple cider vinegar

Apples and apple cider vinegar are loaded with antioxidants. Quercetin is a powerful antioxidant found in apples. Research has shown that quercetin aids with diminishing hot flashes during menopause. Quercetin, the "magic" hot flash food cure helps reduce oxidative stress and damage to cells in the body. Why does this matter? Research has shown a positive connection between high levels of oxidative stress and an increase of menopausal symptoms, especially hot flashes. When midlife women consume apples or apple cider vinegar, the quercetin decreases the intensity of their hot flashes. And unfiltered apple cider vinegar cleans toxins out of the body. This phenomenon has been shown to help decrease sweating, therefore reducing the intensity of hot flashes in midlife women.

4. Menopause Symptom: Osteoporosis

Food Cure = Calcium-rich non-dairy foods/Dark leafy greens

Leafy greens are excellent sources of both calcium and vitamin K. Calcium is needed for bone production, and vitamin K helps regulate calcium to aid with an increase in bone density. "Going green" can reduce the chances of decreased bone density, fractures, and osteoporosis in women experiencing menopause. Dairy is an excellent source of calcium and an important mineral for bone health. Unfortunately, as we transition into the menopausal stage, our midlife bodies tend to be more sensitive to dairy. The good news is there are many calcium-rich non-dairy options to choose from. Some of my favorites include calcium fortified nut milks, such as almond and soy *(do not use soy products if you or anyone in your family has been diagnosed with breast cancer)*. Tofu, raw almonds, and dark green leafy vegetables are also excellent sources of calcium. Dark green leafy vegetables, such as spinach and kale, contain vitamin K, a variety of flavonoids, as well as calcium and have been shown to aid with a reduction in bone loss. In fact, a serving of kale has more calcium than milk!

The Standard American Diet (SAD)

It's no wonder the standard American diet is also known as the "SAD" diet. It is high in processed food. The SAD diet is also high in refined carbohydrates and other chemically laden foods that interfere with how our hormones function. This is especially true during women's midlife years.[7] To feel our best, avoiding processed foods made from white flour, white rice, pasta, and bread products is important. Simple carbohydrates like these raise cortisol levels and elevate blood sugars. This leads to cravings for more of the wrong foods—a vicious cycle. So how do we break the cycle we get ourselves into?

Before you try changing your diet, I recommend a 5-day cleanse. My 5-Day Hormone Reset Cleanse is not a fasting detox. This plan keeps you feeling full and satisfied while cleansing your body inside and out. Before I share the cleanse details, let's talk about some amazing results you may experience from this reset.

Five Significant Results of the 5-Day Hormone Reset Cleanse

1. **Less mood swings:** You will feel positive emotional changes starting day one. Your mood will shift to a more calm and balanced state. This is due to the stabilization of your blood sugars.
2. **Clearing of brain fog:** You will notice you can think more clearly and concentrate better and for longer periods of time.
3. **No more bloating:** From day one, you will notice you are no longer bloated. It flushes the extra fluids and your bowels, which is a main cause of bloating.
4. **Weight loss:** You will lose weight (between two and five pounds is the

average for a 5-day hormone detox reset cleanse).

5. **Clearer skin:** You will notice your skin becomes clear and has a glow to it. This is because of the flushing of toxins from your body and the nutrient-rich foods you are consuming.

Because of my many issues with food during the midlife stage, I have made my midlife transition much easier by creating the 5-Day Hormone Reset Cleanse. The recipes for the five-day cleanse are ones I designed. I complete a full five-day hormone cleanse every one to three months or as needed. The results are astounding. On the first day, I feel less bloated and have more mental clarity, and by day five, I feel thirty years younger!

Please note that I cannot guarantee that everyone will have the same results from this plan, but I can tell you that all of the patients who have been on this plan have reported positive results. The recipes in this book and on my website may contain allergens, which is a unique concern for each individual. If you or anyone you share my recipes with has a food allergy, you may substitute a food item from the same category that will not cause an allergic reaction.

Now that you have read about the four magic foods to help the most common bothersome menopausal symptoms, the SAD diet, and the five results you might experience with the cleanse, it is time for your reset.[8]

Ready, Reset, Go!

Here is your 5-day hormone reset. The smoothie and tonic recipes help to relieve symptoms that come along our menopause journey. These delicious remedies also aid with boosting metabolism, weight loss, increasing energy, and providing an overall glow, inside and out. Enjoy!

Instructions

Follow the plan exactly as it is written for five days. Use the guide to set your goals and preplan. Choose a smoothie from the recipe list as a breakfast and dinner meal. You may substitute one snack per day for one serving of the deep chocolate avocado pudding (dessert). Drinking smoothies and tonics each day accelerates the cleansing process and gets you relief as soon as day one!

This five-day rest will prepare your body for a longer-term change, which we'll dive into a bit later.

---

[1] *Disclaimer: The hormone reset cleanse and lifestyle diet plan in this book is in no way to be used as a substitute for medications or medical advice prescribed by your medical doctor. If you are diabetic or have any chronic medical condition, please speak with your doctor before beginning these or any other changes to your diet. Please note that everyone is unique and may not experience the same relief at the same time.*

5-Day Hormone Reset Plan Guide

Recipes for your 5-day reset plan are set up in three categories:

Tonics: Help you regain hormonal balance and relieve symptoms, such as bloating and hot flashes.

Smoothies: Work alongside the tonics to aid with symptom relief while offering a variety of nutrients. Helps with satiety, decreases cravings, and speeds up weight loss.

Dessert: Allows for variety and aids with decreasing cravings.

5-Day Hormone Reset Cleanse Recipes

TONICS

Tonics are low-calorie liquid boosters used in small doses for medicinal purposes.

1. Apple Cider Hot Flash Tonic

- 8 oz pure filtered water or distilled water
- 2 tablespoons of organic raw apple cider vinegar

- 1 organic cinnamon stick

Directions: Make this tonic each night and keep in a sealed mason jar overnight. Drink upon waking and before bed. *If you are unable to tolerate this tonic, you may use apple cider vinegar on salads as a dressing.

2. Gold Detox Tea

Calms the mind and body and helps prevent bloating.

- ½ of an organic lemon-squeezed into a juice
- ¼ tsp of organic ground turmeric
- 1 pinch of fresh organic ground black pepper
- 6 fresh organic mint leaves (you may use 1 teaspoon of dried mint leaves)
- 1 teaspoon of organic chamomile flowers
- 1 cup of pure filtered water or distilled water
- 1 teaspoon of pure organic maple syrup (optional)

Directions: Bring the filtered water to a boil, then add all ingredients into a tea steeper or a teacup and allow it to sit until the ingredients have settled to the bottom. When tea turns a deep golden color, begin to sip slowly (while observing your morning meditation routine and prior to bedtime).

3. Green Bone Tonic

Keeps your bones strong.

- 1 cup organic spinach
- 1 cup of organic kale
- Juice of 1 organic lemon
- Juice of 1 organic lime
- 1 cup pure filtered water or distilled water
- ½ teaspoon of fresh organic grated ginger
- ¼ teaspoon organic ground turmeric
- ¼ teaspoon of freshly ground organic black pepper

Directions: Add all the ingredients into a blender until it turns into a liquid, you may add water if needed. Store your tonic in a mason jar (write the date on the jar). Drink ¼ cup every morning on an empty stomach. Keep in a sealed dated mason jar, will stay fresh refrigerated for about 3 days.

SMOOTHIES

Smoothies are liquid nutrient-rich drinks that may be substituted for a meal or enjoyed as a snack.

Quick Reset Smoothie Guide

Making a hormone reset-busting smoothie is easy! Be sure to measure: 6 ounces equals a snack, and 12 ounces equals a meal substitute.

Sample Hormone Reset Busting Smoothie

½ cup low-fat organic Greek yogurt (thickener)
½ cup pure filtered ice cubes (liquid)
½ cup organic frozen berries (fruit)
½ cup organic kale (vegetable)
1 level teaspoon organic chia seeds (super charge)

Directions: Add all ingredients into a blender mix and enjoy!!

---

*Or use the following smoothie guide to create your own delicious hormone busting smoothies!

Just combine your preferred organic ingredients from each column of the table on the following page in a blender, then pulse until smooth.

CREATE YOUR OWN SMOOTHIE GUIDE

Fruits	Fruits & Veggies	Liquids (½ to 1 cup)	Thickener (½ cup)	Supercharge (½–1 tsp)
bananas	apples	pure filtered water	ice	peanut butter
mango	pears	almond milk (unsweetened)	low-fat yogurt	almond butter
papaya	kiwi	rice milk (unsweetened)	plain, low-fat Greek yogurt	Cashew butter
pineapple	melon	soy milk (unsweetened)	silken tofu	plant-based protein (50 calories or less)
mixed berries	watercress	coconut milk/water (unsweetened)	chia seeds (1 Tbs)	cinnamon (pinch)
strawberries	spinach	coconut water (unsweetened)	raw oats (1 Tbs)	turmeric (pinch)
blueberries	kale	¼ cup fresh squeezed apple juice with ½ cup pure filtered water	avocado (1/8)	any spice you desire
peaches	cucumber	¼ cup fresh squeezed carrot juice with ½ cup pure filtered water	ground flaxseed (1 Tbs)	cocoa powder

* Note: Use fresh or frozen organic fruits & veggies. Use any fruit or a mix of fruits as long as it's not more than a ½ cup for a snack or a full cup as a meal replacement. Use a measuring cup; don't estimate. Feel free to use as many of the non-starchy vegetables as you'd like and be creative with your options.

If you're not ready to create your own, here are specific recipes you can follow to make delicious smoothies:

1. *Kale-Avocado Breakfast Smoothie*

Helps with weight loss.

- ½ cup low-fat organic plain Greek yogurt
- 1 cup fresh organic spinach
- ½ small frozen organic banana
- ¼ organic avocado
- ¼ cup ice cubes (made with filtered water/distilled water)
- 12 raw organic unsalted almonds (chopped)
- Organic cinnamon

Directions: Combine low-fat Greek yogurt, spinach, banana, avocado, and ice in a blender. Puree until smooth. Sprinkle chopped almonds and cinnamon on top (optional). Enjoy as a breakfast.

Nutrition Facts (Serves 1)
- Calories 298
- Protein 17g
- Carbs 25g
- Fat 17g
- Fiber 7.1g
- Sugar 11g

2. Golden Milk Smoothie

Helps with mood swings.

- Juice of a ¼ of an organic freshly squeezed lemon
- ½ cup organic papaya
- 1 tbsp of organic ground flax seeds
- 1 tsp pure organic vanilla extract
- ½ tsp ground organic turmeric
- Pinch of fresh ground organic black pepper
- ½ cup pure filtered or distilled water or made into ice cubes
- ½ cup unsweetened organic almond milk or organic Greek yogurt
- Pinch of organic cinnamon or nutmeg

Nutrition Facts (Serves 1)
- Calories 144
- Protein 3.5g
- Carbs 17g
- Fat 7.1g
- Fiber 5.2g
- Sugar 9.1g

Directions: Combine all ingredients and mix in a blender until smooth, then sprinkle with cinnamon and nutmeg and enjoy!

3. Super Bone Strengthening Smoothie

Help keep bones strong.

- 1 cup raw organic greens (kale, spinach, any green you desire)
- ½ small ripe banana (frozen if you prefer)
- 2 teaspoons raw organic almond butter
- 1 tablespoon fresh squeezed organic lime or lemon juice
- ½ cup organic low-fat Greek yogurt
- ½ cup filtered ice cubes
- 4 fresh mint leaves
- Cinnamon, nutmeg, or turmeric for garnish

Nutrition Facts (Serves 1)
• Calories 182
• Protein 14g
• Carbs 18g
• Fat 7g
• Fiber 3g
• Sugar 11g

Directions: Put all ingredients into a blender. Sprinkle with above spices and almond meal with fresh mint leaves and enjoy anytime!

DESSERTS

1. Deep Chocolate Avocado Pudding

Helps curb cravings and helps prevent weight gain

- ¼ of a ripe organic avocado
- 1 organic date (pitted and chopped)
- ½ teaspoon vanilla extract
- ½ cup organic Greek low-fat yogurt
- 2 teaspoons unsweetened organic cocoa powder
- ¼ cup of organic mixed berries

Nutrition Facts (Serves 2)
- Calories 206
- Protein 15g
- Carbs 19g
- Fat 11g
- Fiber 9.4g
- Sugar 6.5g

Directions: Add all of the ingredients to a blender and mix until smooth. Put the pudding into two glasses and chill in the refrigerator. Top with fresh berries and enjoy!

General Instructions for the
5-Day Hormone Reset

Remember, this is a five-day plan that will prepare your body and mind for a longer-term change we'll discuss soon.

1. Three (3) meals per day (breakfast smoothie, lunch meal, dinner smoothie).
2. Two (2) snacks per day (you may substitute 1 serving of the delicious deep chocolate avocado pudding for one daily snack—see recipe).
3. Drink pure filtered water or distilled water upon waking and throughout the day, before and after meals, for a total of sixty-four (64) ounces per day minimum (ideal is ½ your body weight in ounces).
4. You may enjoy organic herbal tea made with pure filtered water anytime you wish!
5. Limit your fruit to mixed berries (1 measuring cup).
6. Only use organic mixed leafy greens (2 or more measuring cups, the more the better!)

7. Make sure fresh fruits and vegetables are organic and washed well.
8. You may enjoy organic free-range chicken breast or your choice of wild-caught fish for lunch.
9. My go-to lunch is to throw all lunch ingredients into a bowl and make a delicious, chopped salad (you will need a salad knife chopper and a stainless-steel bowl).
10. Drink gold detox tea first thing in the morning and before bed.
11. Drink your green bone tonic sixty (60) minutes after your breakfast smoothie.
12. Enjoy two (2) squares of organic 95 percent dark chocolate (you can have one square during the day and one as an evening snack).
13. No food at least three (3) hours before bedtime.
14. Leave a twelve- to fourteen-hour timeframe between your after-dinner snack and breakfast.
15. Sip on the apple cider hot flash tonic as needed
16. Use the one-day example for your five days (choose any smoothie in the recipe

section for your breakfast and dinner meals).

17. For best results, use measuring cups and spoons.
18. For optimal results, only eat and drink what is on the 5-day reset plan for five days; no substitutes unless you are allergic to something.

Avoid

1. Sugar, honey, stevia, and all natural and artificial sugars.
2. Dairy, except organic low-fat Greek yogurt.
3. Caffeine.
4. Processed food.
5. Artificial ingredients.
6. Eating out.
7. Fast food.

It's time to share a sample menu based on the information you just learned.

5-Day Hormone Reset Sample One-Day Menu

TIME	SAMPLE MEAL
Upon waking	Gold detox tea
Breakfast	Smoothie (see recipe section)
Sixty (60) minutes after breakfast smoothie	Green bone tonic
Lunch	• 6 oz grilled organic wild grilled salmon • 2 teaspoons extra virgin organic olive oil • 2 or more measuring cups of organic mixed greens •
Snack	• 1 cup organic berries • 20 raw organic unsalted almonds
Dinner	Smoothie (see recipe section)
Snack	2 squares of organic, 95% cacao dark chocolate
Thirty to sixty (30–60) minutes before bed	Gold detox tea
Throughout the day	Sip on apple cider hot flash tonic

The Meno*PAUSE* Hormone-Reset Lifestyle Plan

Now that you have completed the 5-Day Hormone Reset Cleanse, it's time follow the **5 Reset Rules** for life and change your eating habits forever. You do not need to count calories, but you should be aware of your food choices and preparation methods. Grilling, baking, air frying, and stir frying are the best low-calorie food preparation methods.

5 Reset Rules for Life

Rule #1	Drink your smoothie within 30–60 minutes of waking *(waking time may vary)*.
Rule #2	After your first meal (see rule #1), eat every 2–4 hours throughout the day. • Eat dinner no later than 3 hours before bed. • If you're hungry after your last meal (dinner), have an evening snack (carbohydrate with a protein).
Rule #3	Always combine carbohydrates (grains, starches) with protein. • With the meal OR on an empty stomach OR with your evening snack
Rule #4	Exercise portion control. • Use the palm of your hand for measuring for weight loss. • Measure up to the end of your pinky for maintenance. • Use your whole hand for measuring while recovering from stress or when you need extra calories or nutrients (ex: after surgery).

	• Use one small or medium plate for your meals. • Always think in this size order for portion control: • Veggies: largest part of the meal. • Protein: next largest part of the meal. • Carbs: smallest part of the meal.
Rule #5	Drink plenty of water. • 6–8 oz. glasses or more (unless fluid restriction apply). • Only drink water or seltzer (sodium free). • No juices or sugary beverages (liquid calories count as food!). • Avoid sugar-free beverages (artificial sweeteners are not healthy and increase or cause menopausal symptoms).

MenoPAUSE Hormone Reset Dietary Guidelines
(For a Lifelong Change)

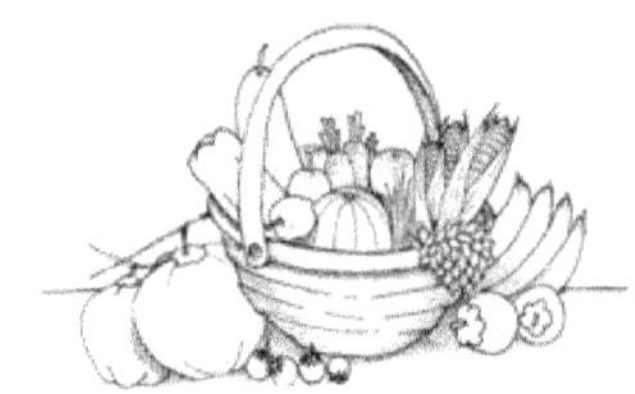

1. Drink 8 to 12 eight-oz glasses of pure filtered water each day. (1 glass upon waking, 1 glass before and after each meal, 1 glass or more in the evening and before bed)
2. Drink herbal tea: mint, ginger, or turmeric (do not add sugar or any sweeteners).
3. Use an organic spray oil for cooking.
4. Eat no more than 1–2 small fresh fruits per day
5. Stick to organic foods.
6. Eat wild fish, grass-fed lean beef, and free-range chicken breast.
7. Base lunch and dinner on fresh salads and lean protein.
8. Enjoy a smoothie as a meal replacement. You will feel great and get better results by having a smoothie for your breakfast

meal and avoiding bread, rice, and pasta while choosing a starchy vegetable instead of a carb.

9. Have an organic hardboiled egg as a substitute snack.

10. Leave 12 hours between your last meal and your morning meal.

Avoid

- Sugar, honey, stevia, and all artificial sugars
- Simple carbohydrates
- Artificial ingredients
- Dairy, except organic low-fat Greek yogurt
- Caffeine
- Processed food
- Eating out (particularly fast food)

The Meno*PAUSE* Hormone Reset Food Groups

Below is a mini guide to ensure you are eating from each food group while adapting a hormone-reset lifestyle. The foods listed below are the best hormone-busting foods to help relieve menopausal symptoms. Please visit my website for more options.

Grains/Starches	Whole grains, starchy vegetables (80 calories per serving).
Proteins	• Fatty fish, lean meats, and poultry (55 calories per oz, 4–6 oz per meal, 220–330 calories). • Nuts (6–12 pieces, 45–90 calories). • Seeds (45–90 calories). • Nut butters (2 level teaspoons, 110 calories per serving).
Dairy	Low-fat Greek yogurt, Kefir (plain organic yogurt rich in probiotics) (1 cup, 90–120 calories).
Fats	• Olive oil (1 teaspoon, 45 calories) • Avocado (1/8, 45 calories). • nuts, seeds (see protein).
Fruits	Fresh organic fruits (choose the smallest or 1 measuring cup worth of mixed fruit).
Vegetables	Non-starchy organic vegetables (unlimited, add a minimum of 2 measuring cups worth to lunch and dinner).

Purchase organic products when possible. Enjoy something from each food group each day and make this a lifelong reset plan!

THIRTY DAYS TO A NEW YOU

For the next thirty days, track how your body feels and any changes you notice while using these new meal plans. To start the thirty-day routine, complete the mood chart below. Rate your current mood on a scale of 1–10, with 10 being extremely negatively impacted by the symptom, and 1 indicating that symptom is not an issue affecting your life right now. Then, at the end of the thirty days, there is another worksheet to complete. You might by surprised by the changes you feel!

Mood	On a scale of 1–10 how much does each symptom negatively impact your daily life since you have made changes to your diet?
Anxiety	
Crying Spells	
Depression	
Difficulty Concentrating	
Insomnia	
Irritability	
Lack of Motivation	
Mood Swings	
Sadness	
Tiredness	

Now you're ready to begin. Use the sample meal plan below and the recipes for smoothies and tonics in this book as guides to help guide you with creating a thirty-day meal plan. You may check out my website for more recipes www.nutritionist4u.com.

Meno*PAUSE* Hormone Reset Sample Day

Breakfast

3 egg whites (protein)
spinach (veg)
onions (veg)
tomato (veg)
1 teaspoon of organic extra virgin olive
oil (fat)
½ cup cooked plain organic steel oats made
with pure filtered water (grain)
Or a smoothie (see smoothie guide and
recipes in this book and on my website)

Lunch

4–6 oz grilled organic wild Salmon
(protein)
mixed organic leafy greens, red, yellow,
and green peppers (veg)
2 teaspoons extra virgin organic olive
oil (fat)
juice of ½ organic lemon (free)
1 small organic sweet potato (starchy veg)

Snack

1 small organic green apple (fruit)
2 teaspoons natural organic almond butter
(fat)
Or an organic free range hard-boiled egg
(protein)

Dinner

4–6 oz grilled organic free range grilled
chicken breast (protein)
steamed organic broccoli (veg)
organic mixed greens (veg)
2 teaspoons organic extra virgin olive
oil (fat)
2 teaspoons Braggs aminos (free)
½ cup cooked organic quinoa (grain)

Snack

4 plain 100% whole grain crackers (grain)
2 teaspoons organic almond butter (fat)

Now that you started making permanent changes to your eating habits, it's time to track your food and mood.

Activity: Track Your Food and Mood

At the end of the thirty days, use the worksheet below to rate your mood relief on a scale of 1–10, with 10 being extremely negatively impacted by the symptom, and 1 indicating that symptom is not an issue affecting your life right now. Compare your ratings to the chart you filled out before initiating the thirty-day meal plan.

Mood	On a scale of 1–10 how much does each symptom negatively impact your daily life since you have made changes to your diet?
Anxiety	
Crying Spells	
Depression	
Difficulty Concentrating	
Insomnia	
Irritability	
Lack of Motivation	
Mood Swings	
Sadness	
Tiredness	

Visit my website, www.nutritionist4u.com, for additional recipes and sample meal plans.

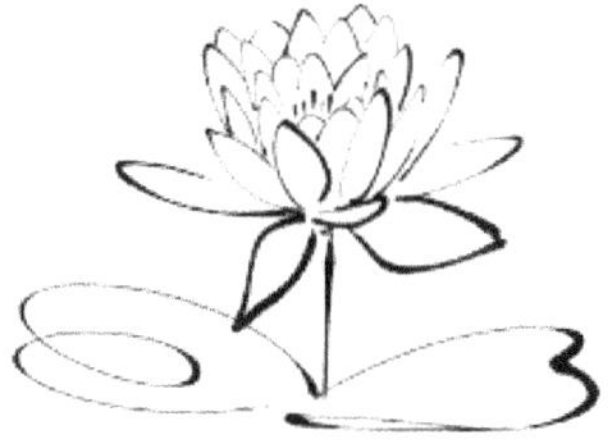

The Guest House

This being human is a guest house.
Every morning a new arrival,
A joy, a depression, a meanness,
some momentary awareness comes
as an unexpected visitor.

Welcome and entertain them all!

Even if they are a crowd of sorrows,
who violently sweep your house,
and empty it of its furniture,
still, treat each guest honorably.

He may be clearing you out
for some new delight.
The dark thought, the shame, the malice—
meet them at the door, laughing, and invite them in.

Be grateful for whatever comes
because each has been sent

as a guide from beyond.

~ Jellaludin Rumi[9]

. . .

"The Guest House" was written by thirteenth-century Persian poet Jalāl-ad-Dīn Rumi. The main purpose of this poem is to remind us not to resist thoughts and emotions that come to our minds, but to accept them with courage, kindness, and respect.

Chapter 8
MOVEMENT MATTERS

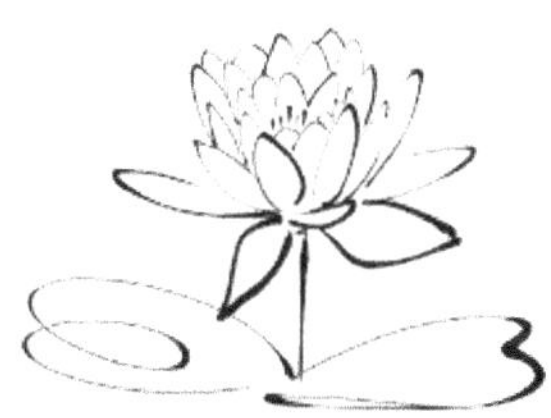

For women going through menopause, regular physical exercise is essential.[1] Our movement matters. No, you don't need to run a marathon or begin CrossFit, but you should get into a habit of adding physical activity to your daily routine to take good care of your body. After all, you only get one, and it is as Rumi says, "A guest house."

According to the Mayo Clinic, there are several reasons fitness is important during menopause:

1. Preventing weight gain.

> *Around menopause, women tend to lose muscular mass and increase belly fat. Regular physical exercise might assist you in avoiding gaining weight.*

I remember looking through my parents' photo album (in those days we had albums. I am sure you remember that!). I saw a photo of myself at age two. The funny—or should I say shocking—thing was that fat was rolling over my shoes. Most people would say it was cute, but that "cute" fat stayed with me throughout my life.

At the age of twelve, I tried my first diet. My cousin told me that she went on the "Scarsdale Diet." To me, my cousin always looked like a model, and I didn't understand why she'd go on a diet. I wanted to look like my cousin, so I begged her to show me the diet plan. I tried it but couldn't last for a day.

I wasn't very big; I was what people called, "chubby." As the years went by I gained and lost weight, trying numerous diets. At age fourteen, I decided I had enough of dieting and being labeled "chubby." I became aware of my food intake and drank only water. I also joined a gym, "Elaine Powers," and went four times a week after school. I started to lose my chubbiness and felt better about myself. After a few months, I contacted Ford Modeling Agency. During my interview, they told me that I would have gotten a contract if I was a year younger or older. I was too short for the adult division and too old for the kids' division. I wasn't very upset because I was in awe that a modeling agent from Ford would even speak to me.

A few weeks after that meeting, I signed with a manager and started booking movies, commercials, and print ads. I was even in a film with Harvey Keitel (he told me I had "beautiful lips!"). I was on the road to stardom, or so I thought.

At the age of eighteen, I met a young man who would become my husband within seven months (we are still married to this day!). I had my first child at nineteen. She was born prematurely at twenty-eight weeks. This is why I lost the "baby weight" right after birth. At twenty years old, I had my second child after gaining about seventy pounds during my pregnancy. That time, I had a hard time losing the weight.

When my second child was six months old, I joined a gym, and boy was I upset when the gym manager asked if I was pregnant! I worked hard to lose the baby weight, eating healthy foods and exercising on a regular basis. I lost weight and felt amazing.

Then at ages thirty-one, thirty-three, and thirty-five, I had three more kids. At that point, I was not gaining as much weight as I did with my second pregnancy, but it became harder to get it off my older body.

At age thirty-seven, I finally achieved my goal weight and kept it off. I found a running routine —but by no means was I "a runner." I ran out of desperation. I bought a book and followed the guide and was able to do two short runs of five miles each, then build up to long runs of twelve miles. I felt amazing, but then I got that job, where I had the long commute—twelve to sixteen hours dedicated to work, five days a week.

I stopped my running routine, and the weight came back. Perimenopause began to kick in. I decided to be reasonable, so I joined a yoga studio and went after work two or three times a week. On weekends, I either ran, swam, or biked. I loved yoga and meditation so much that I became a certified instructor. I realized that to keep my weight in a good place and feel great, I had to set a reasonable schedule, which included rest time as well. This is how I found the *PAUSE* Formula.

2. Reducing the risk of cancer.

Exercise can help you lose weight or maintain a healthy weight during and after menopause, which is protective against cancers, such as breast, colon, and endometrial cancer.[2,3]

3. Strengthening your bones.

After menopause, exercise may help reduce bone loss, reducing the risk of fractures and osteo-porosis.[4]

Case Study

Lidia a fifty-three-year-old woman was diagnosed with osteopenia prior to seeking out my services. Lidia stopped her exercise routine because of her fear of breaking a bone. She slowly gained weight and became more susceptible to bone fractures. I explained to Lidia that staying physically active and getting daily exercise are especially important for midlife women during the transitional years. I came up with a weekly exercise schedule for Lidia, and not only did she lose weight, but her osteopenia improved, helping her avoid osteoporosis in the long term.

If you have been told by your doctor that you already have bone loss, you should stick with low-impact weight-bearing exercises because of the risk of fractures. The best way for keeping midlife bones strong and healthy is to include weight-bearing and muscle-strengthening exercises. Weight-bearing exercises include low- and high-impact exercises where you push against gravity. Below are examples of high- and low-impact exercises and muscle strengthening activities to keep your bones strong.

4. Reducing the risk of other diseases.

Weight gain during menopause could have major health consequences, increasing risk for multiple diseases. [5]

Overweight people are more likely to develop heart disease and Type 2 diabetes. Regular exercise can help to mitigate these risks. Such is true with June, a fifty-eight-year-old woman who was interviewed and said, "Menopause forced me to exercise more. Once I hit fifty, I had to because I had to be one step ahead."

5. Boosting your mood.

Adults who engage in physical activity have a decreased incidence of depression and cognitive deterioration.[6]

For me physical activity is an emotional outlet for stress. It is therapeutic when I challenge my body with exercise. I often begin my workouts in stress mode, but once I get into it, I feel amazing. Exercise, meditation, and yoga help clear my mind and relax my body. A relaxed mind and body are the formula to health and happiness.

One of my patients, Anna, once told me that exercise not only keeps her in shape but gives her confidence to take on daily tasks. It reminds her that her body can do more than she ever realized. Anna stays focused and grounded as she keeps up with her three-day-a-week exercise routine. She also mentioned her weight and bloating issues as well as hot flashes had almost "disappeared" after a month of regular exercise. Anna feels better than she ever did in her now fifty-four-year-old body.

Another patient, Diana, stated, "With the guidance from Dr. Renata, my dietitian, I was able to lose weight during menopause. When I lost my first ten pounds, I went to the grocery store and picked up a ten-pound bag of rice and carried it around to remind me how much weight I had been [lugging]. I knew that losing weight would make me feel better, and it did. I started as a pre-diabetic, then all of my numbers normalized. I not only felt good about myself, but my stomach felt better too. Maintaining an active lifestyle became very important to me because not being active is not living. I find joy in being physically active and like to stay active with dancing. I love salsa dancing, and I also go for walks with my sister."

Activity: Do Something Physical

I encourage you to think about how you can add exercise into your weekly routine. If you are currently active, think about how you can change up your activity to reap even more benefits from exercise.

Weight-bearing and muscle-strengthening exercises, such as cardio, running, and speed walking have numerous benefits. These types of activity help to decrease body fat, increase lean muscle, which supports the joints, aids with balance, and most of all, high-impact activities help build bones that are thicker and stronger, decreasing the likelihood for fractures.

Use the list below to get ideas of which exercises you would enjoy and add one or two a minimum of three to four times a week for thirty to sixty minutes. *(Please make sure you are cleared by your doctor before beginning any new exercise routine.)*

Low-Impact Weight-Bearing Exercises	<ul><li>Low-impact cardio</li><li>Yoga</li><li>Swimming</li><li>Walking</li><li>Stair climbing</li><li>Gardening</li><li>Elliptical machine</li><li>Stepper machine</li><li>Hiking</li><li>Slow dancing</li></ul>
High-Impact Weight-Bearing Exercises	<ul><li>High-impact cardio</li><li>Speed walking</li><li>Jogging</li><li>Running</li><li>Jumping rope</li><li>Hiking</li><li>Dancing</li><li>Treadmill</li><li>Tennis</li><li>Zumba</li></ul>

Muscle-Strengthening Exercises	<ul><li>Lifting weights (free weights or machines)</li><li>Resistance band exercises</li><li>Intensive outdoor gardening</li><li>Climbing stairs</li><li>Walking up a hill</li><li>Biking</li><li>Non-stop dancing at a fast pace</li><li>Sit-ups</li><li>Squats</li><li>Push-ups</li><li>Any exercise which uses your own body weight as resistance</li></ul>
General Exercise	<ul><li>Cardio: 30-60 minutes of cardio, 3-4 times per week (must be cleared by doctor, adhere to individualized plan)</li><li>Weight training (includes weight-bearing exercises)</li><li>Light stretching (includes yoga)</li></ul>
The Daily to-do's	<ul><li>Read food ingredients: *"If you can't read it, don't eat it!"*</li><li>Exercise: Cardio four or more times a week for 30–60 minutes.</li><li>Walk: Daily goal is 10,000 steps.</li><li>Keep a food/mood/symptom diary.</li></ul>

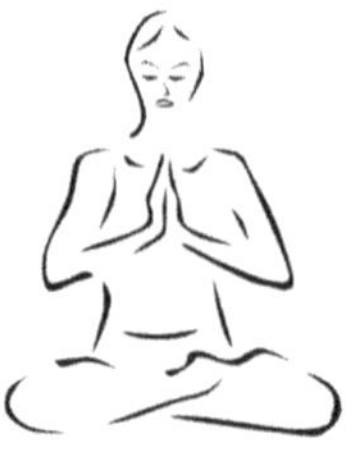

JOURNAL BREAK

A Time to *PAUSE* and Reflect

Get cleared for exercise with your doctor, then choose one exercise you would like to begin and create a plan for how to incorporate it into your week.

____

____

____

____

____

____

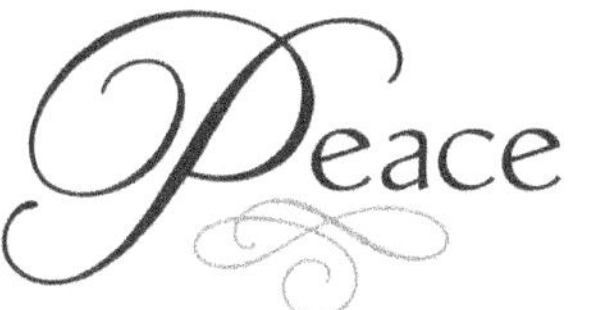

Chapter 9
YOGA & MEDITATION FOR MENOPAUSE

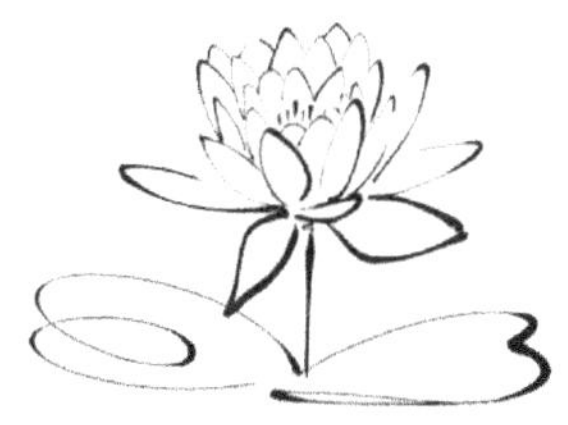

Yoga and Meditation

Yoga and meditation fill my heart and soul.
They are the things that make me feel whole.
Yoga and meditation are dear to me.
Yoga and meditation make my mind and body free.

~ Dr. Renata

Yoga and meditation are key to relieving emotional and physical menopausal symptoms.[1] The midlife women I have counseled over the years—especially the ones who have been members of my "Menopause Mama's Club"—report experiencing "miraculous relief" from the dreaded *"M"* symptoms. Their *"M"* relief is not only due to healthy changes in the diet but occurs because of their ongoing practice of yoga and meditation.[2] This is by no means a complete cure for all of the symptoms midlife women experience. The sixteen women surveyed for this book reported at least 95 percent relief from their *"M"* symptoms. They also said they began to enjoy their daily lives again when keeping up with their newfound lifestyle. This is mostly true when midlife women adapt to a regular ongoing yoga and meditation practice, which calms the body and mind, relieving many of the uncomfortable symptoms connected to menopause.

Yoga and meditation are beneficial for managing numerous menopausal symptoms, such as pain and stress.[3,4] Consider how your body normally reacts to menopausal symptoms: your stomach and digestive system may be uncomfortable on a regular basis; your emotions may be awry; your mind may feel cloudy, or you may have difficulty sleeping. Yoga can help with the emotional side effects of menopause as well as the physical discomfort.

Restorative yoga necessitates holding positions for longer periods of time than traditional yoga, frequently with the use of props such as folded blankets to help the body rest. The nervous system is calmed by these positions. While there are several different types of yoga and meditation out there, I will share specific successful techniques that I have used in the past for myself and my patients.

The breath, otherwise known as *pranayama* or (controlled) breathing, is a powerful tool and a key to that relief. When we breathe correctly, our breath alleviates negative feelings, thoughts, and desires and quiets the mind and body.[5] Calming the mind and body regularly is why adaptation takes places and we remain calm even when not practicing.

Engage in your yoga and meditation practice a minimum of three times each week, skipping a day to rest between each practice. Eventually, anxiety, mood swings, sleep issues, elevated blood pressure, and other menopausal symptoms improve.

There are numerous styles of yoga and meditation to choose from. Having a varied practice allows for better outcomes.[6] For example, restorative yoga is a practice in which the body is at total rest and relaxation throughout the entire routine. *Vinyasa* is a more rigorous routine that tones muscles and burns calories. Varying your yoga and meditation practice will not only help keep you from being bored but may also be beneficial for relieving close to all forty menopausal symptoms.

My Menopause Yoga and Meditation Story

I love yoga and meditation, not only because of the miraculous relief they offer, but for many other reasons too—too many to list. I had always dreamed of trying yoga but was afraid that I wouldn't be good at it. I was worried I was too old and couldn't twist and turn my body into a pretzel or be able to do a headstand. I learned and built up my body to do most of the twists and turns. But to this day, I still can't do a headstand (I think I am still afraid), but it doesn't matter! I was also worried about how I would look in a yoga outfit and didn't feel comfortable being barefoot.

One day, on my forty-fifth birthday, my daughter gave me a birthday present: a yoga pass for three months. I happened to have some time on my hands to use that pass. It took me a few weeks to get the courage to call the studio and set up my session. On the first day, as I walked closer to the yoga studio, I worried about the things I mentioned earlier. Am I too fat? Too clumsy? Too weird looking? Too old? The fear enveloped me, yet I decided to be brave and go in. After all, it can't be worse than going to the doctor.

I trudged up the stairs and smelled delightful incense burning, causing a pleasant and calming feeling to come over me. I saw a few people who looked amazing, like models and professional yogis. I repeated the affirmation, "You are you and nothing can stop you from the happiness you deserve." I walked courageously to the desk and signed in. To my surprise, everyone was super nice and welcoming. The lady at the desk showed me the studio entrance and told me to take a seat wherever I felt comfortable. As I walked in, I told myself I should sit next to the biggest, clumsiest woman I could find, but I realized that person might be me! So instead, I sat close to the door in case I wanted to quietly "slip" out. To my surprise, once the class began, I forgot my fears, allowing the amazing beauty and essence of the yoga studio to take over. I was one with the amazing model-like yogis. Ever since that first class, I have made yoga and meditation a huge part of my life and cannot imagine my life without it.

Below are forty reasons why I am in love with yoga and meditation. (I chose forty—though there are too many to count—because forty aligns with the forty most common and dreaded *"M"* symptoms.)

40 Reasons I Love Meditation and Yoga

1. Anyone, any age, with any body type or shape, can practice them.
2. Provide inner peace.
3. Offer ways to relax and de-stress.
4. Help me manage my mood swings.
5. Minimize my hot flashes.
6. Lower my blood pressure and heart rate.
7. Help with bloating.
8. Maintain a healthy weight.
9. Keep me flexible.
10. Alleviate muscle pain.
11. Alleviate joint pain.
12. Alleviate back pain.
13. Boost my self-esteem.
14. Encourage me through self-expression.

15. Inspire me.
16. Balance my life.
17. Calm my body and mind.
18. Give me something to look forward to.
19. Keep me in a happy state.
20. Make me feel powerful,
21. Give me strength.
22. The yogis are super nice people.
23. Make me feel beautiful.
24. Keep my mind sharp.
25. Lessen my fatigue.
26. Keep my anger at bay.
27. Help me see the positives in all situations.
28. Make me a better human being.
29. Keep me feeling alive.
30. Can be modified to my body.
31. Help me sleep better.
32. There is no pressure from others in the classes.
33. There are many styles to match my mood.
34. Create a place for an escape from reality.
35. Keep me vibrant in my body and mind.
36. Keep me looking young.
37. Great for glowing skin.
38. Offer the ability to practice with like-minded women.

39. Allow me to feel like a "glam-ma" rather than a grandma.
40. Practicing yoga and meditation can become a lifetime routine no matter what age you are!

Bottom line: Do something you enjoy. Empty your mind of negativity. Take an "alone time out", fifteen to twenty minutes of "me" time daily.

- Meditation (practice for 5–10 minutes upon waking and at bedtime)
- Walk, read, dance, find a hobby

Another Success Story

"Dr. Renata has always encouraged me to go further and do better, and it's the faith she has in me, sometimes when I don't even see it in myself. She's the best. I don't know anyone else that just cares about everyone that way. She makes time for me; I can call her right now and say, 'I have to talk to you,' and she will listen and give me the best advice. She supports me in every part of my life. Dr. Renata showed me how yoga and meditation can change it, and they have changed me.

She made me realize that the symptoms will pass. I feel a lot better now, and the meditation helps a lot. I really saw improvement after I changed my eating habits and lifestyle choices. I will always remember Dr. Renata's positive attitude, compassion, humbleness, and how wise she is."
~*Angelica*

Meditation & Mindfulness

Earlier, we talked about taking a *PAUSE*. Meditation is actually a form of pausing. It's not necessarily just sitting in silence for a long time, but it's purposeful thinking and relaxing. Sometimes, our minds are racing from worry or because we feel overwhelmed. Whatever the cause, mindful meditation can help.

I love yoga and meditation so much that at the age of fifty-five, I became a certified yoga and meditation instructor. Yoga and meditation have not only given me the gift of health and vitality, but the gift of the practice has also given me a chance to help other midlife women realize their bodies—like mine—are gifts to use and treasure always.

I was never confident or flexible, and I always felt awkward, especially when it came to team sports and group exercise. Through my yoga and meditation practice, I became more flexible and stronger in my body and mind. Not only did I notice amazing changes in my body, but my mood stabilized, and I was able to live each day in a positive manner. The gifts of yoga and meditation gave me an inner awakening like no other. In fact, since I have been a practicing instructor, I have experienced a mental and physical clarity like never before. My muscle and joint pain are minimal, my brain fog is gone, and my concertation has greatly improved. I could not have written this book during my "*M*" years without having a grounding meditation practice.

Try the following deep breathing meditation exercise to help relieve your stress and symptoms of menopause:

Activity: 6-4-8 Meno*PAUSE* Reset Breathing Technique

6-4-8 BREATHING[7]

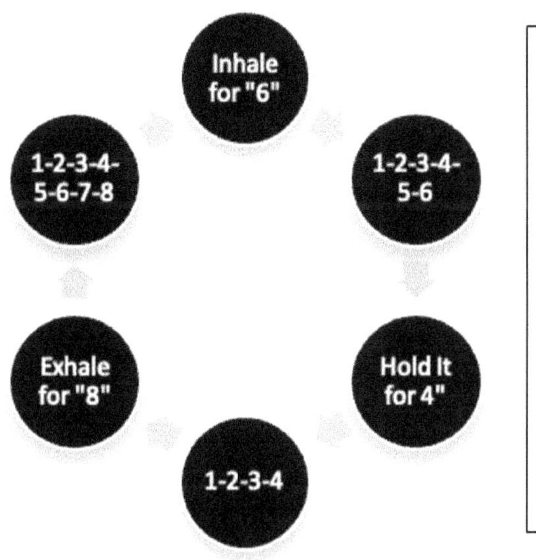

Sit in a comfortable position (either in a chair or on a yoga mat).

Starting with the inhale, follow the arrows.
⇒ Breathe in for a slow count of 6 through your nose, filling your lungs.

⇒ Hold it for a count of 4.

⇒ Breathe out through your mouth for a slow count of 8.

*Always make the exhale a little slower than the inhale. This calms the body and mind.

Yoga for Menopause Symptom Relief

Using gentle yoga as a form of relief for menopausal symptoms allows the body and mind to remain calm, creating balance and inner and outer strength between the two.[8]

I have chosen three yoga poses (*asanas*), which are my go-to "cure" when I am in immediate need of relief. Feel free to modify these yoga poses and use a blanket or blocks to aid with knee pain or as an extra source of comfort. These, and most yoga poses, can be modified and performed seated in a sturdy chair.

1. Cat/Cow Pose

This asana is a blend of two poses, which allow gentle movement within the spine. This creates a gentle opening of the chest while in a cow position and a gentle stretch in cat position. These fluid moves between cow and

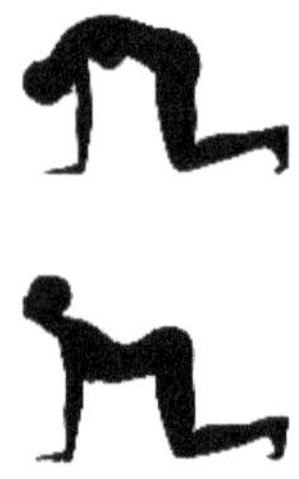

cat massage the joints and tissues around the spine, relieving pain.

Directions:

1. Begin on your hands and knees.
2. Bring your wrists directly under your shoulders.
3. Line up your knees directly below your hips.
4. Spread your knees equal to the width of your hips.
5. Inhale and tuck your toes.
6. Expand your chest forward (engage your abdomen keeping your spine neutral).
7. Exhale, relaxing the tops of your feet.
8. Round your back through your lower spine.
9. Relax your head and take a few deep 6-4-8 breaths.

Forward Facing Hero's Pose

This modified hero's pose truly makes you feel like a menopausal hero. This is because of the lowering of your head beneath your heart, the gentle stretching of your inner thighs, and the relaxing stretch of the spine, all which allow calm, peace, and joy to enter your body to relieve numerous symptoms.

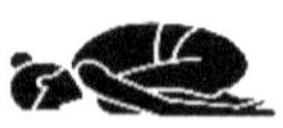

Directions:

1. Sit on your knees on a mat, carpet, or blanket.
2. Place your knees as far apart as feels comfortable.
3. Make sure your heels are apart and your big toes are touching.
4. Sit on your heels.
5. Lengthen your tailbone down toward the floor, being sure to keep your spine long.
6. Gently bring your hands forward or keep them at your sides; fully extending your spine and gently gliding your shoulder blades onto your back.
7. Keep your arms and hands shoulder-width apart.
8. Relax your forehead onto the floor and keep your neck nice and long.

9. Take three deep, cleansing breaths and slowly release.

Legs-Up-the-Wall Pose

This stress-relieving pose allows all of the muscles in the body to completely re-lax, reducing stress and anxiety while gently stretching the hamstrings and chest. Please note: You can use a blanket, blocks, or a cushion to alleviate back pain.

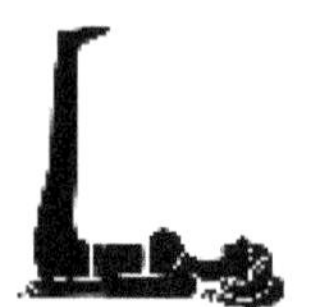

Directions:

1. Place a folded blanket or cushion and the short edge of a yoga mat against a wall to support your hips.
2. Lay down with your head and shoulders on your mat and your hips on the folded blankets, then slowly and gently raise your legs and place them against the wall.
3. You can move a little further away from the wall or closer to the wall to feel comfortable.
4. Take a deep breath and close your eyes while gently moving your chin to your

Chapter 10
COMPLEMENTARY & ALTERNATIVE TREATMENTS (CAM)

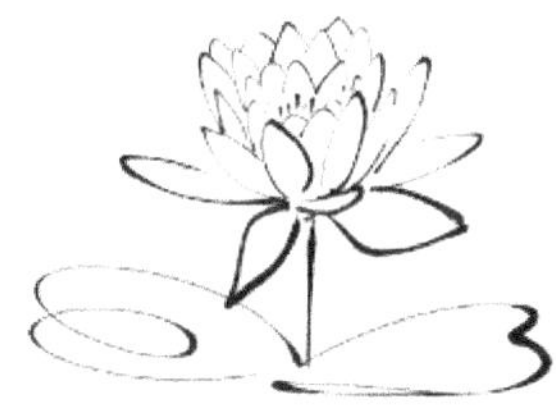

What are alternative and complementary treatments?

Complementary therapy refers to treatments used *alongside* traditional medical approaches to treating symptoms. Complementary therapy "complements" traditional medical treatment.[1] **Alternative therapy** is used *in place of* traditional medical approaches.

What are the benefits of complementary and alternative therapies?

Complementary and alternative therapies target specific issues related to symptoms. These therapies help relieve the symptoms of menopause, such as stress, anxiety, pain, bloating, and hot flashes.[2]

Why am I sharing these CAM therapies?

Nontraditional therapies have become widely used, even in conventional medical settings. Over the years, numerous studies on various alternative and complementary therapies for menopausal symptoms have proven them to be a safe method of helping to relieve bothersome menopausal symptoms. Though the therapies throughout this book may be used as complementary or alternative treatments for menopausal symptoms. The three therapies I mention in this chapter (chakra healing, Reiki, and essential oil healing) may not be for everyone and are less often utilized, yet they are safe and have credible mechanisms of action.[3]

1. Chakra Healing and Menopause Relief

Chakras provide "spiritual energy" for our bodies. They help optimize the function of our organs as well as our minds. There are seven chakras in the body, and each one has a purpose.

The sacral chakra, *Svadhishthana,* is situated in the pelvic area just below the naval. This chakra is connected to our desires and emotions and emits the color orange. A blocked sacral chakra causes an increase in menopausal symptoms.[4,5]

A blocked sacral chakra may contribute to:

1. Disinterest
2. Seclusion
3. Worry
4. Anxiety
5. Loneliness
6. Low libido
7. Loss of creativity

Practicing meditation and relaxation assists with opening blocked chakras. Chakra yoga is a form of yoga practice which combines a variety of yoga styles which in combination help to stimulate the bodies energy centers (*chakras*). This form of yoga combines meditation with various yoga poses (asanas) and includes breathing techniques and mantra chants to release blockages.[6,7]

2. Reiki and Menopause Relief

As a certified Usui Shiki Ryoho Reiki practitioner, I would be remiss not to include a few notes about it. After all, I want to ensure you enjoy a long, healthy life, it is the only one you have!

Usuai Shiki Ryoho Reiki, which I practice, was founded by Dr. Mikau Usui. This form of Reiki honors the lineage of Mikao Ususi, Chujiro Hayashi, Hawayo Takata, Phyllis Lei Furumoto, and Johannes Reindl.

The practice of Reiki is recognized by The National Center for Complementary and Alternative Medicine (*NCCAM*) as biofield energy therapy. Biofield energy consists of magnetic and electrical fields formed through living organisms, such as the human body. The heart, brain, and every cell in the human body produce electrical currents to function. In Reiki, energy is transferred through the light touch of the practitioner's hands. Touch is the exchange of magnetic fields, which stimulates all the systems in the body and explains the seemingly miraculous outcomes of Reiki for women experiencing menopausal symptoms.[8,9,10,11,12,13]

Not only does reiki offer healing, but it also helps calm the mind and thought patterns. In Reiki, there are principles similar to the Yamas and Niyamas in yoga. These principles are known as *precepts,* which help to purify mental and emotional bodies. Precepts refer to the moral and ethical principles by which one lives.

Below are the five precepts of Reiki for health and well-being[14]:

1. Just For Today, Do Not Worry

2. Just For Today, Do Not Anger

3. Honor Your Parents, Teachers And Elders

4. Earn Your Living Honestly

5. Show Gratitude To Every Living Thing

~ Dr. Mikao Usui

3. Essential Oils and Relief

Aromatherapy uses scents released from essential oils to activate the hypothalamus, a part of the brain that influences hormones. Smell affects mood, metabolism, and stress level.

There are several essential oils that could be used to alleviate many menopausal symptoms. Make sure you use pure organic essential oils.[15] *Never ingest essential oils.*

These are my two favorite "go-to" oils:

Lavendar: Add a few drops of lavender oil to a cold compress and place it on an area of discomfort. Diffusing lavendar oil may help relax you and can be used as a sleep aid.[16]

Peppermint: Add a few drops of peppermint oil to a cold compress and place it on an area of discomfort. You may also inhale peppermint oil for relaxation.[17]

Chapter 11
FEEL LIKE YOURSELF AGAIN

I Am Me

I am not you; I am me,

I am worthy, I feel free.

I am happy, I am joyful,

I am proud, and I am soulful.

I am not my past; I am not my future,

I am the present and who I was meant to be!

~Dr. Renata

Menopause can bring on a flurry of changes that sometimes feel endless. There was a time I thought my symptoms would go on forever. I wondered if I would ever feel like myself again. I had no idea that I could feel better than I did before, and you can too!

Hopefully, after going through the various activities in this book, you feel better already . . . maybe almost "normal." It may seem as though you will never feel completely normal again after menopause. Please take my story and the stories of the many women mentioned in this book and use them as inspiration for what is possible for you.

You can enjoy life!

You can be happy!

You can reduce menopausal symptoms!

You *can* feel like yourself again!

In reality, once actual menopause is reached, you will not only feel "normal" again, but you will also have a beautiful, rejuvenated feeling of self and life vitality. Most women feel even younger than they did before the *change*.

Take a Picture and Enjoy Your Life

It is said, "Like a photograph, life isn't made in the bright moments. We develop from all the negatives. It takes darkness and challenges to reveal the beauty underneath." I know this to be true. While life's challenges, including the unpleasant experiences associated with the "*M* word" may seem to cast shadows over our lives, I urge you to reassess. Take another look and recognize that we are similar to a photograph in that we develop from negatives as well. We are evolving into better versions of ourselves, even when circumstances seem dark. Just as the photography process makes the picture sharper, allowing the image's real beauty to shine through when it comes into contact with light, the same thing happens to us as we navigate menopause. We become the best versions of ourselves! Your best days are ahead of you and not behind you, so get ready.

June, one of the sixteen midlife women interviewed for this book, has a positive attitude when it comes to menopause and getting older. When asked, "In what ways has life gotten better post-menopause?" June answered, "It shouldn't be taboo; it's not the old lady disease. You don't have to be set in your life. It should be natural process. It's like a pebble in my shoe—not a big deal. That is the message I want girls to know. It's something nice to look forward."

I, like June, have also adapted a healthy outlook on menopause. I feel younger than ever and enjoy a vibrant lifestyle. On January 18, 2021, I became a grandma to a beautiful baby girl named Lucy Renata (yes named after me). Wait! Did I say grandma? I meant glam-ma! Yes, you read it correctly I am like a grandma but way more fun and fabulous! Menopause won't stop me from enjoying life. It won't ruin the fun times spent with my granddaughter. I want many more years of fun and enjoyment as a "glam-ma." I want to stay vibrant and enjoy my life to the fullest. Keeping up with my *PAUSE* Formula lifestyle is the key.

Take a Pause

As this book comes to a close, take a moment to *PAUSE* and consider all that has been covered thus far. Utilize what you've learned to help you succeed as you move into the next chapter of your life. Complete the final two exercises below, and if you still need encouragement or a supportive group, please visit my website for information on how to stay connected: www.nutritionist4u.com.

Activity: What Do You See?

What do you see when you look at yourself in the mirror? Do you see how beautiful you are? Do you notice how much wiser you are? Do you see a woman with a bright future?

Without even looking at you physically, I can tell you that you are beautiful because you are unique. You are wise because of all that life has taught you, and your future is bright because you are stepping into the best years of your life. For this activity, answer these questions on the next few journal pages, using as much detail and emotion as needed:

- What do you see when you look in the mirror? Be as descriptive as possible.
- What one word would you use to describe yourself? Why that word?
- What have you learned about yourself while reading this book?

- If given thirty minutes on a stage to speak to women ten years younger than you, what advice would you give?

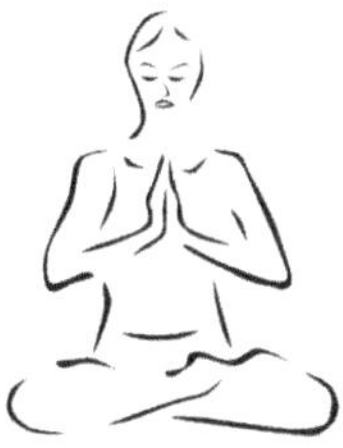

JOURNAL BREAK

A Time to *PAUSE* and Reflect

What do you see when you look in the mirror? Be as descriptive as possible.

____

____

____

____

____

____

____

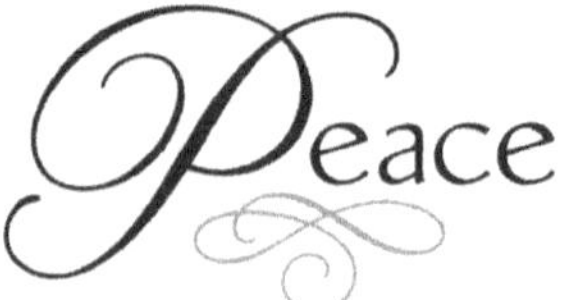

What one word would you use to describe your-self? Why that word?

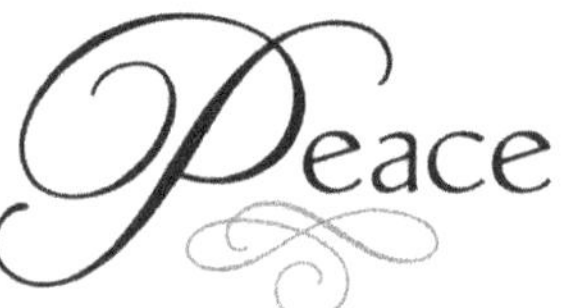
Peace

What have you learned about yourself while reading this book?

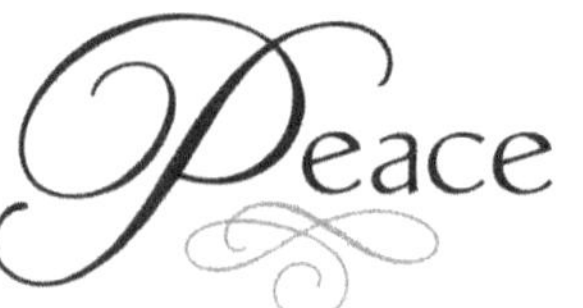
Peace

If given thirty minutes on a stage to speak to women ten years younger than you, what advice would you give?

____

____

____

____

____

____

____

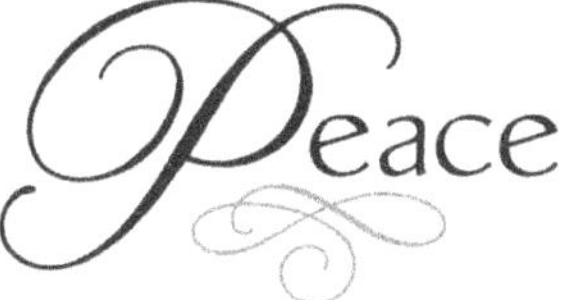

Peace

Chapter 12
THE FUTURE YOU

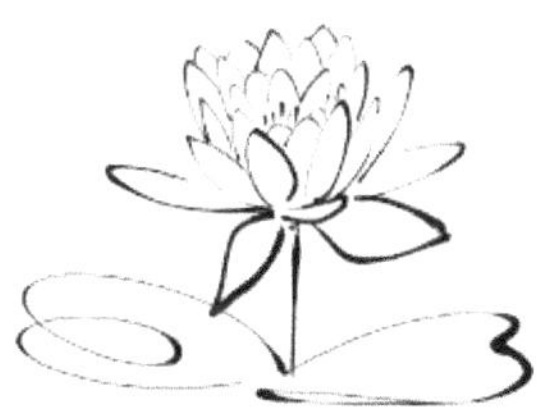

When you think about your life one, five, or even ten years down the road, what do you see? Are you enjoying life? Do you see yourself happy?

Without being a person who can predict the future, I am a person who can use past successes to make assumptions about what could be. Therefore, I can tell you that you can enjoy your life. You can have more fun now than you did in your twenties and thirties. You can be happy regardless of what happens. Take a moment to answer in detail the questions in the following journal break.

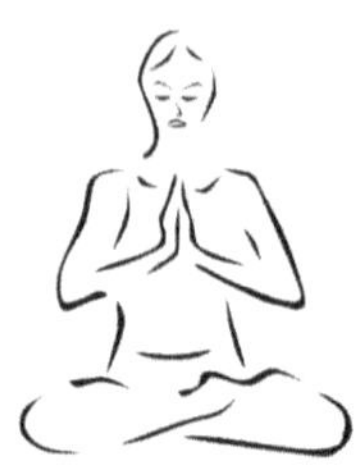

JOURNAL BREAK

A Time to *PAUSE* and Reflect

What *one word* would you use to describe your future? Why that word?

____

____

____

____

What do you see when you imagine your future? Be as descriptive as possible.

____

____

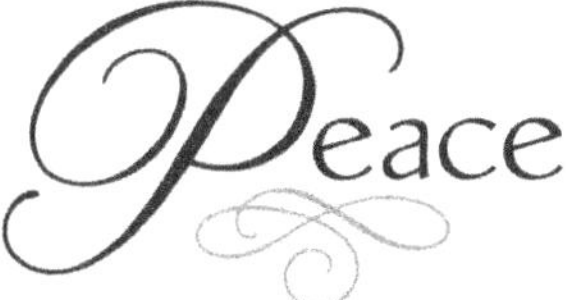

What lesson will you have learned from going through menopause?

____

____

____

____

____

____

____

____

____

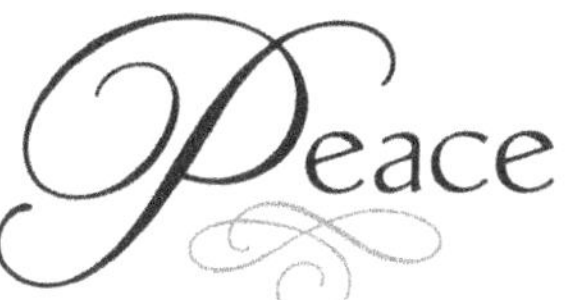

Peace

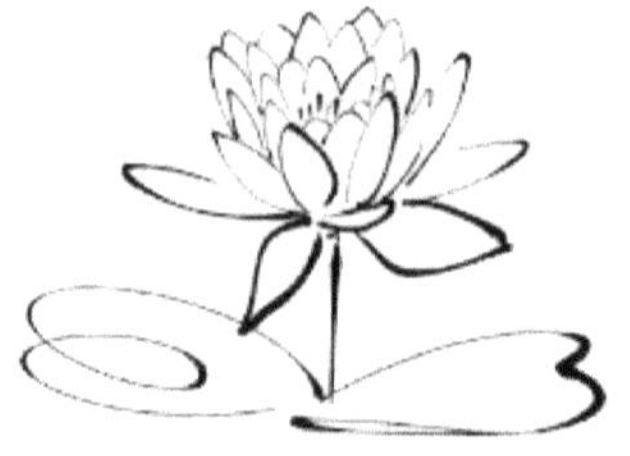

You Should

You should not fear, for fear is fruitless.

You should not dread, for dread never transpires.
You should not panic, for panic is insignificant.

You should not borrow other people's problems,
for other's problems clutter your happiness.
You should not let others bring you down,
for it interferes with positive thoughts.

You should sleep with a clear mind,
for a clear mind makes a noble bedfellow.
You should restore the past, whether good or ill,
before it is gone forever.
You should count your blessings,
for they can vanish before your eyes.
You should listen, for only when you listen do you hear.

Most of all,
You should appreciate YOU!!

~ Dr. Renata

A Final Note To My Fellow Menopause Warriors

During my younger days, I had never heard the word *menopause*. I was not informed or educated about this transitional journey. Because of a lack of knowledge and support, I, too, was not prepared for my transitional journey.

This led to dark days, where I didn't leave the house or my bed and spent thousands of dollars on treatments that worsened my symptoms.

My personal menopausal journey was a rough one, but as I say, "Everything bad is for something good." I used my experience to help other midlife women end their needless suffering and live the lives they deserve.

Women are warriors and should not have to suffer the way I did. Physicians, family members, friends, and employers should be educated about just how debilitating menopause can become. The lack of education and awareness is the main reason women suffer with their health and well-being, in their careers and relationships.

It is also time to make menopause education and awareness a priority in health classes and for medical students as part of their curriculum. This can help to inform family, friends, employers, and others and ensure autonomy for midlife women.

Now that you have read my book, I hope you feel better and have found peace and hope in your midlife journey. I am your "Menopause Mentor," so you, too, can be a "Menopause Warrior!"

- Check out my website, www.nutritionist4u.com, for resources and support.
- Join my Menopause Facebook group: Nutritionally Speaking with Dr. Renata, Your Menopause Mentor, and meet fellow menopause warriors.

Let's win this battle together because you are never alone as a fellow menopause warrior!

Additional Resources

If you want to learn more about menopause, please utilize the resources below, which are meant to supplement the content found in this book.

> www.ncoa.org/article/why-menopause-matters
> www.menopause.org
> www.womenshealth.gov/menopause
> www.imsociety.org
> www.nationalmenopausefoundation.org
> www.redhatsociety.com

The Future Is the Present

My life to me is dear,
Yet there is hesitation and fear.
I want to be loved,
I want to be free,
Most of all, I want to be me.
I cry, I shout, I take a breath,
I let it out.
I am a woman, I am free.
The future is the present to me.

~ Dr. Renata

Acknowledgments

There are always many people to thank, and I do so with so much gratitude. To my dietetic interns and volunteers, who did a great deal of research, interviewed the sixteen women who were kind enough to share their stories, and assisted with the recipes and scientific information. I hope this experience has taught you that the sky is the limit, and no matter what situation you may be in or how hard life may be, you can achieve anything you desire if you do not give up. I encourage all of you to take your careers to the highest limits and beyond.

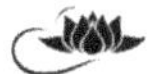

I want to especially thank Kim Vargas and Suzette Negron, who worked many months—even on their off time—to help with research, interviews, organization, and ideas. To all my students over the years, you've been a blessing.

An extended thank you to Suzy Rosenstein, my life coach, and her "Women in the Middle" group. Suzy, your encouragement and wisdom gave me the inspiration and strength to put my pen to the paper and begin writing this book. You helped me to become a stronger person due to your ongoing support and camaraderie. Through your program I have learned to appreciate my "midlife" years and have become more resilient than I have ever been.

A very special thank you to Shara Hutchinson, without whom this book would not have been possible. Thank you for allowing me to tap into your brilliant mind. Thank you for your support, hard work, and dedication. Thank you for listening to me ramble on and on and stopping me in time to gather my thoughts. I will always remember what you taught me: "Done is better than perfect . . ." because ". . . perfection is achieved when nothing needs to be taken away."

A heartfelt thank you to Danielle Barry, the kindest person with the purest soul. And to Laura Lapierre, my best friend since childhood, one of the most selfless and caring people you'll ever meet. Both gone too soon but kept in my heart, always.

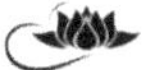

Thank you to my group and one-on-one patients —my dedicated fellow menopause warriors. And thank you to the ladies from my "Wellness Wednesday Workshop." I love you all.

To the sixteen women who permitted me to document part of their menopausal journeys in this book. I appreciate you. I hope it gives you comfort to know you are serving others. (In alphabetical order) Angelica, Anna, Carmen, Diana, Debbie, Francis, Janet, Jenny, June, Krystal, Letty, Lidia, Marisol, Norma, Pam, Patresse.

To my friends and colleagues, Dr. Amie Hornaman and Dr. Jessica Tischenial - thank you. I have learned so much throughout our doctorate journey. You allowed me to ease out of the conventional world and find my way into the world of functional and integrative nutrition through your kindness, generosity, support, and friendship.

To my friends from childhood and beyond, thank you for your encouragement and for always supporting me in all I do. Thank you for your advice and lending me your ears when I needed someone to listen to me. Thank you for long nights of crying on your shoulders, and most of all, thank you all for always making me feel like there is nothing I can't do, cheering me on when I am down, and for your lifelong friendships.

To Leigh, my fellow bestie, whom I met in a peri-menopause group on Facebook years before the big "M", though we have never met in person, we have gone through this journey together, supporting each other along the way.

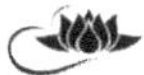

To Anu Butani, of Reiki of Long Island, you have changed the way I view my daily life and the world. Thank you for your Reiki offerings, your kindness, and helping to awaken my spirituality.

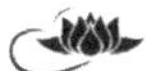

To my loving family, especially the women, in the USA, Israel, Czech Republic, and England, especially Lily. Thank you to my five amazing children: Daniella, Micky, Teddy, Jonathan, and Benjamin - whom all understand the hormonal issues Daniella and I have suffered with. I want to thank you from the bottom of my heart for allowing me to "runaway" for many weekends to achieve deadlines. Thank you for putting up with my schedule during my doctorate studies and for the duration it took to write this book. I want you to know that I appreciate each one of you and love you to the moon and back. I want to especially thank my husband Eli for sleeping in an empty bed all those nights while I wrote this book, and for understanding (and dealing with) my PMS, perimenopause, and menopause all these years. I appreciate you and your support. I love you.

An extra special thanks to my beautiful granddaughter Lucille (Lucy) Renata. Lucy, you were born during the birth of this book. You are pure joy, and you give me happiness and always make me smile. I promise to guide you, so you never have to experience any PMS, perimenopausal, and menopausal symptoms the way I did. I love you with all my heart forever and ever; "Just me and you forever, yeah!" Of course, I cannot forget my grand-dogs, Artie and Edith.

Lastly, a very special thank you to my mother, Jarmila, who was my best friend in life and will always be my eternal best friend. You suffered in silence and never complained about your menopausal symptoms. To my father, Theodore, you were the strongest and smartest person I've ever known; you taught me to overcome life's obstacles. I dedicate my doctoral degree to you. And to my brother, Peter, may you live a happy and healthy life. My entire family, I keep you all in my heart and as we used to say, *kamaradi,* which means "friends" in Czech. Our heart strings will always be tied together.

About the Author

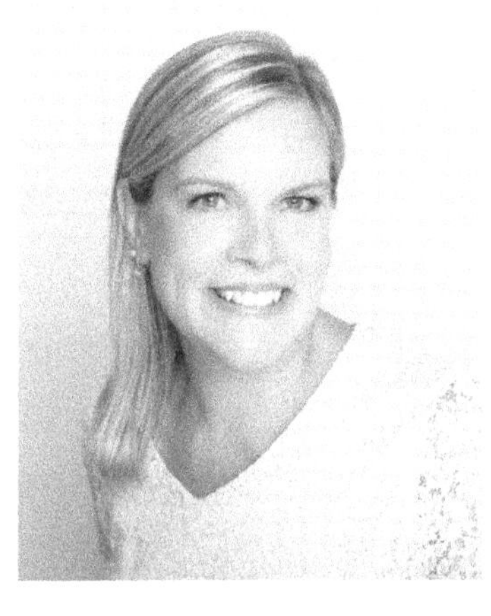

Dr. Renata Shiloah, DCN, MS, RD, CDN, RYT, CMT, is an accomplished and passionate Doctor of Clinical Nutrition and Integrative Health with over twenty years' experience. She is also a certified yoga and meditation teacher and certified Usui Shiki Ryoho Reiki practitioner. Dr. Renata practices Reiki, honoring the spiritual lineage of Mikao Usui, Chujiro Hayashi, Hawayo Takata, Phyllis Lei Furmoto and Johannes Reindl. She served as the director of the nutrition department at outpatient clinics as well as an adjunct professor in the Health Sciences Department at Lehman College, CUNY.

Before receiving her Doctoral Degree from Maryland University of Integrative Health, she earned a Bachelor of Arts degree in family, nutrition, and exercise science from Queens College CUNY and a Master of Science degree in Healthcare Policy and Management and Nutrition from Stony Brook University Medical Center, which led her to becoming a registered dietitian.

Dr. Renata, as she is commonly called, has been featured in numerous magazines and publications, including *Teen Vogue, Prevention, SHAPE, American Dietetic Association Journal, Fitness Magazine*, and the *Daily News*. She's appeared on "Good Morning America" and UPN Channel 9 News "I-Team" and was a nutrition spokesperson for Channel 12 News. In addition to her various certifications and accreditations her wellness programs have received best practice recognition from the Health Resources and Services Administration and the American Board of Bariatric Medicine.

She welcomes new members to her Facebook group, Nutritionally Speaking with Dr. Renata, Your Menopause Mentor.

Dr. Renata was born in Prague, Czech Republic, and arrived in New York City with her family at age four. She enjoys spending time with her husband, five children, and her beautiful granddaughter. Her favorite activities, to no surprise, include yoga, meditation, swimming, bike riding, and power walking.

You can find her at www.nutritionist4u.com.

Appendix

Medicinal plants can be a healthy way to conquer some of the most common menopausal symptoms. Though supplements may be beneficial and safe for some during menopause, as we have discussed throughout this book, the safest way to help relieve your menopausal symptoms is with nutrition, yoga, and meditation, which are what I'd rather see readers use to relieve their symptoms.

For informational purposes, I have included eight common and relatively safe supplements, which have been shown to relieve some menopausal symptoms in midlife women. Please be advised that these may have adverse effects and may interact with certain medications. Use common sense and speak with your medical doctor before taking these or any over-the-counter supplements.

8 Supplements to Try for Menopausal Symptoms

Supplement	Possible Benefits	Possible Adverse Effects	Warnings
Black Cohosh	Relieves hot flashes, night sweats, insomnia, mood disorders, and headaches	Nausea, mild skin rash	Do not take if you have a history of liver disease
Evening Primrose Oil	Lessens severity of hot flashes	Nausea, stomach pain	Interacts with some HIV medications
Flax Seeds	Reduces hot flashes; aids with bone health	May cause stomach cramping (increase amount slowly over time)	Considered safe

Maca	Increases sex drive, reduces vaginal dryness, and lessons depression/anxiety	No significant adverse effects have been documented	Do not take if you have a family history of or have had a hormone-related cancer
Probiotics	Relieves bloating, constipation	Upset stomach, diarrhea, cramping	Immune-compromised individuals should not use due to risk of infection
Red Clover	Reduces hot flashes and night sweats	Headache, nausea, weight gain	Do not use for more than twelve (12) months; do not use if pregnant of breastfeeding or if you have a history of breast or any other hormone-related cancer
Soy	Lessens hot flashes; aids with bone health	Stomach pain, diarrhea	Do not take if you have a family history of or have had a hormone-related cancer
Valerian	Calms the mind and body, reduces insomnia and hot flashes	Upset stomach, headaches, drowsiness, dizziness	Do not take with medications for sleep issues or anxiety; interacts with kava, St. John's wort, and melatonin

Endnotes

References for General Content

Gabriela Pichardo, MD. (2020, May 25). "Menopause." Retrieved from WebMD, https://www.webmd.com/menopause/guide/menopause-basics.

George, S. A. (2002). "The Menopause Experience: A Woman's Perspective." *Journal of Obstetric, Gynecologic, and Neonatal Nursing: JOGNN, 31*(1), 77–85, https://doi.org/10.1111/j.1552-6909.2002.tb00025.x.

Mayo Clinic. (2019, October 16). "Embracing A Positive Mindset During Menopause From Mayo Clinic." Retrieved from Thorne, https://www.thorne.com/take-5-daily/article/embracing-a-positive-mindset-during-menopause-from-mayo-clinic.

Mayo Clinic Staff. (2021, March 12). "Fitness Tips for Menopause: Why Fitness Counts." Retrieved from Healthy Lifestyle, https://www.mayoclinic.org/healthy-lifestyle/womens-health/in-depth/fitness-tips-for-menopause/art-20044602.

Mohamad Ishak, N. N., Jamani, N. A., Mohd Arifin, S. R., Abdul Hadi, A., & Abd Aziz, K. H. (2021). "Exploring women's perceptions and experiences of menopause among East Coast Malaysian women." *Malaysian Family Physician: The Official Journal of the Academy of Family Physicians of Malaysia, 16*(1), 84–92, https://doi.org/10.51866/oa1098.

Nelson, J. (2021, May 12). "The Best Diet to Reduce Menopause Symptoms." Retrieved from The Checkup, https://www.singlecare.com/blog/menopause-diet/.

Smith, M. (2021, December 4). "25 Encouraging Words of Affirmation for Women." Retrieved from 95.5 The Fish, https://955thefish.com/content/family/words-of-encouragement-for-women-45-affirmations-to-lift-the-soul.

Sussman, M., Trocio, J., Best, C., Mirkin, S., Bushmakin, A. G., Yood, R., Friedman, M., Menzin, J., & Louie, M. (2015). "Prevalence of Menopausal Symptoms among Mid-Life Women: Findings from Electronic Medical Records." *BMC Women's Health*, *15*, 58, https://doi.org/10.1186/s12905-015-0217-y.

The Association for Women's Health Care. (2021, December 4). "How Menopause Affects Your Mental Health." Retrieved from The Association for Women's Health Care, https://www.chicagoobgyn.com/blog/how-menopause-affects-your-mental-health.

Traci C. Johnson, MD . (2021, August 9). "The Emotional Roller Coaster of Menopause." Retrieved from WebMD, https://www.webmd.com/menopause/guide/emotional-roller-coaster.

What Is Menopause? | National Institute on Aging. (n.d.). Retrieved June 20, 2022, from https://www.nia.nih.gov/health/what-menopause.

References for 5-Day Cleanse Recipes

Becker, S. L., & Manson, J. A. E. (n.d.). *"Menopause, the gut microbiome, and weight gain: correlation or causation?" Menopause: The Journal of The North American Menopause Society.* Retrieved November 21, 2021, from https://journals.lww.com/menopausejournal/Fulltext/2021/03000/Menopause,_the_gut_microbiome,_and_weight_-gain_.14.aspx?casa_token=_TTVbTdzPEkAAAAA%3AQy-Mp_KO9kM-

53YA8arXutFGfMgkk2JhFQXWy7Dd9Ee5nuFPkpAav-NinnhFCWrkekRs0bF095NTtG0sEeQoIPjSw.

Fulgoni III, V. L., Dreher, M., & Davenport, A. J. (n.d.). "Avocado consumption is associated with better diet quality and nutrient intake, and lower metabolic syndrome risk in US adults: Results from the National Health and Nutrition Examination Survey (NHANES) 2001-2008." *Nutrition Journal.* Retrieved November 21, 2021, from https://pubmed.ncbi.nlm.nih.gov/23282226/.

Hewlings, S., & Kalman, D. (2017). "Curcumin: A review of its effects on human health." *Foods*, *6*(10), 92. https://doi.org/10.3390/foods6100092.

Kulkarni, S. K., Bhutani, M. K., & Bishnoi, M. (2008, September 3). "Antidepressant activity of curcumin: Involvement of serotonin and dopamine system." Psychopharmacology. Retrieved November 21, 2021, from https://link.springer.com/article/10.1007%2Fs00213-008-1300-y.

MediLexicon International. (n.d.). "Menopause and anxiety: What is the link?" Medical News Today. Retrieved November 19, 2021, from https://www.medicalnewstoday.com/articles/317552.

Naidoo, U. (n.d.). *"Eat to beat stress."* SAGE *Journal.* Retrieved November 20, 2021, from https://journals.sagepub.com/doi/full/10.1177/1559827620973936.

Ware, M. (n.d.). *"12 health benefits of avocado."* Medical News Today. Retrieved November 21, 2021, from https://www.medicalnewstoday.com/articles/270406#benefits.

Zhu, L., Huang, Y., Edirisinghe, I., Park, E., & Burton-Freeman, B. (2019). "Using the avocado to test the satiety effects of a fat-fiber combination in place of carbohydrate energy in a breakfast meal in overweight and obese men and women: A randomized clinical trial." *Nutrients*, *11*(5), 952. https://doi.org/10.3390/nu11050952.

References for Tonics and Smoothies

Brennan, D. (2020, November 3). "6 foods high in quercetin and why you need it." WebMD. Retrieved November 20, 2021, from https://www.webmd.com/diet/foods-high-in-quercetin#1.

Doshi, S. B., & Agarwal, A. (2013, July). "The role of oxidative stress in Menopause." *Journal of Mid-Life Health.* Retrieved November 20, 2021, from https://www.ncbi.nlm.nih.gov/pmc/articles/PMC3952404/.

References for Yoga and Meditation

Vaze, N., et al. *Journal of Mid-Life Health, 1.* 2010;2:56–58.

Laughlin-Tommaso, SK. https://www.mayoclinic.org/diseases-conditions/high-blood-pressure/expert-answers/menopause-and-high-blood-pressure/faq-20058406.

Bankar, MA, et al. *J Ayurveda Integrative Med.* 2013;4(1):28–32.

Warner, S. E., & Shaw, J. M. (2000). "Estrogen, Physical Activity, and Bone Health." *Journal of Physical Education, Recreation & Dance, 71*(6), 19–23. https://doi.org/10.1080/07303084.2000.10605156.

Cramer H, Peng W, Lauche R. Yoga for menopausal symptoms- A systematic review and meta-analysis. Maturitas. 2018 Mar;109:13-25. doi: 10.1016/j.maturitas.2017.12.005. Epub 2017 Dec 6. PMID: 29452777.

References for Appendix (Supplements)

Kargozar R, Azizi H, Salari R. A review of effective herbal medicines in controlling menopausal symptoms. Electron Physician. 2017 Nov 25;9(11):5826-5833. doi:

10.19082/5826. PMID: 29403626; PMCID: PMC5783135.

The North American Menopause Society. "Nonhormonal management of menopause-associated vasomotor symptoms: 2015 position statement of The North American Menopause Society." *Menopause*, 2015;22:1155–72.

Farzaneh, Farah & Fatehi, Setare & Sohrabi, Mohammad-Reza & Alizadeh, Kamyab. (2013). "The effect of oral evening primrose oil on menopausal hot flashes: A randomized clinical trial." *Archives of Gynecology and Obstetrics*. 288. 10.1007/s00404-013-2852-6.

Chen LR, Ko NY, Chen KH. „Isoflavone Supplements for Menopausal Women: A Systematic Review." *Nutrients*. 2019 Nov 4;11(11):2649. doi: 10.3390/nu11112649. PMID: 31689947; PMCID: PMC6893524.

Kargozar R, Azizi H, Salari R. "A review of effective herbal medicines in controlling menopausal symptoms." Electron Physician. 2017 Nov 25;9(11):5826–5833. doi: 10.19082/5826. PMID: 29403626; PMCID: PMC5783135.

Geller SE, Studee L. "Botanical and dietary supplements for menopausal symptoms: what works, what does not." *J Women's Health* (Larchmt). 2005 Sep;14(7):634–49. doi: 10.1089/jwh.2005.14.634. PMID: 16181020; PMCID: PMC1764641.

Szydłowska I, Marciniak A, Brodowska A, Loj B, Ciećwież S, Skonieczna-Żydecka K, Palma J, Łoniewski I, Stachowska E. Effects of probiotics supplementation on the hormone and body mass index in perimenopausal and postmenopausal women using the standardized diet. A 5-week double-blind, placebo-controlled, and randomized clinical study. Eur Rev Med Pharmacol Sci. 2021 May;25(10):3859-3867. doi: 10.26355/eurrev_202105_25953. PMID: 34109594.

Abdi F, Alimoradi Z, Haqi P, et al. "Effects of phytoestrogens on bone mineral density during the menopause transition: a systematic review of randomized, controlled trials." *Cli-*

macteric. 2016;19(6):535–545.

Ghazanfarpour M, Sadeghi R, Roudsari RL, et al. "Red clover for treatment of hot flashes and menopausal symptoms: a systematic review and meta-analysis." *Journal of Obstetrics and Gynaecology.* 2016;36(3):301–311.

Kanadys W, Baranska A, Jedrych M, et al. "Effects of red clover *(Trifolium pratense)* isoflavones on the lipid profile of perimenopausal and postmenopausal women—A systematic review and meta-analysis." *Maturitas.* 2020;132:7–16.

National Institutes of Health, "Valerian", accessed August 2, 2022, https://ods.od.nih.gov/factsheets/Valerian-Health-Professional/#ref.

Shin BC, Lee MS, Yang EJ, Lim HS, Ernst E. "Maca (L. meyenii) for improving sexual function: a systematic review." BMC Complement Altern Med. 2010 Aug 6;10:44. doi: 10.1186/1472-6882-10-44. PMID: 20691074; PMCID: PMC2928177.

Levis S, Griebeler ML. "The role of soy foods in the treatment of menopausal symptoms." J Nutr. 2010 Dec;140(12):2318S-2321S. doi: 10.3945/jn.110.124388. Epub 2010 Nov 3. PMID: 21047930; PMCID: PMC2981010.

Cetisli NE, Saruhan A, Kivcak B. "The effects of flaxseed on menopausal symptoms and quality of life." Holist Nurs Pract. 2015 May–Jun;29(3):151–7. doi: 10.1097/HNP.0000000000000085. PMID: 25882265.

References for Marked Endnotes

Preface

1. Vaze N, Joshi S. Yoga and menopausal transition. J Midlife Health. 2010 Jul;1(2):56-8. doi: 10.4103/0976-7800.76212. PMID: 21716773; PMCID: PMC3122509.
2. Johnson A, Roberts L, Elkins G. Complementary and Alternative Medicine for Menopause. J Evid Based Integr Med. 2019 Jan-Dec;24:2515690X19829380. doi: 10.1177/2515690X19829380. PMID: 30868921; PMCID: PMC6419242.

Introduction

1. Marlatt KL, Pitynski-Miller DR, Gavin KM, Moreau KL, Melanson EL, Santoro N, Kohrt WM. Body composition and cardiometabolic health across the menopause transition. Obesity (Silver Spring). 2022 Jan;30(1):14-27. doi: 10.1002/oby.23289. PMID: 34932890; PMCID: PMC8972960.

2. WIN THE FIGHT AGAINST MENOPAUSE

1. Oakwood Theme Park, "What Does It Feel Like to Ride a Roller Coaster?" (Sept 30, 2019), accessed August 2, 2022, https://www.oakwoodthemepark.co.uk/blog/sin-cat egoria/what-does-it-feel-like-to-ride-a-

rollercoaster/#:~:text=It%20feels%20like%20y-ou%20are,%2C%20fear%20and%20pure%20heav-en%E2%80%80%9D.

2. "The Emotional Roller Coaster of Menopause," Web MD, accessed August 2, 2022, https://www.webmd.com/menopause/guide/emotional-roller-coaster.

3. THE MENOPAUSE MINDSET

1. Dweck CS, Yeager DS. Mindsets: A View From Two Eras. Perspect Psychol Sci. 2019 May;14(3):481-496. doi: 10.1177/1745691618804166. Epub 2019 Feb 1. PMID: 30707853; PMCID: PMC6594552.

2. Albert PR. Why is depression more prevalent in women? J Psychiatry Neurosci. 2015 Jul;40(4):219-21. doi: 10.1503/jpn.150205. PMID: 26107348; PMCID: PMC4478054.

3. Nosek M, Kennedy HP, Beyene Y, Taylor D, Gilliss C, Lee K. The effects of perceived stress and attitudes toward menopause and aging on symptoms of menopause. J Midwifery Womens Health. 2010 Jul-Aug;55(4):328-34. doi: 10.1016/j.jmwh.2009.09.005. PMID: 20630359; PMCID: PMC3661682.

4. Conversano C, Rotondo A, Lensi E, Della Vista O, Arpone F, Reda MA. Optimism and its impact on mental and physical well-being. Clin Pract Epidemiol Ment Health. 2010 May 14;6:25-9. doi: 10.2174/1745017901006010025. PMID: 20592964; PMCID: PMC2894461.

5. Wu G, Feder A, Cohen H, Kim JJ, Calderon S, Charney DS, Mathé AA. Understanding resilience. Front Behav Neurosci. 2013 Feb 15;7:10. doi: 10.3389/fnbeh.2013.00010. PMID: 23422934; PMCID: PMC3573269.

6. Bromberger JT, Kravitz HM. Mood and menopause: findings from the Study of Women's Health Across the Nation (SWAN) over 10 years. Obstet Gynecol Clin North Am.

2011 Sep;38(3):609-25. doi: 10.1016/j.ogc.2011.05.011. PMID: 21961723; PMCID: PMC3197240.

7. Kravitz HM, Colvin AB, Avis NE, Joffe H, Chen Y, Bromberger JT. Risk of high depressive symptoms after the final menstrual period: the Study of Women's Health Across the Nation (SWAN). Menopause. 2022 Jul 1;29(7):805-815. doi: 10.1097/GME.0000000000001988. PMID: 35796553; PMCID: PMC9268212.

8. Soares CN. Depression and Menopause: Current Knowledge and Clinical Recommendations for a Critical Window. Psychiatr Clin North Am. 2017 Jun;40(2):239-254. doi: 10.1016/j.psc.2017.01.007. Epub 2017 Mar 6. PMID: 28477650.

9. Files JA, Ko MG, Pruthi S. Bioidentical hormone therapy. Mayo Clin Proc. 2011 Jul;86(7):673-80, quiz 680. doi: 10.4065/mcp.2010.0714. Epub 2011 Apr 29. PMID: 21531972; PMCID: PMC3127562.

10. Vigesaa KA, Downhour NP, Chui MA, Cappellini L, Musil JD, McCallian DJ. Efficacy and tolerability of compounded bioidentical hormone replacement therapy. Int J Pharm Compd. 2004 Jul-Aug;8(4):313-9. PMID: 23924704.

11. Chmouliovsky L, Habicht F, James RW, Lehmann T, Campana A, Golay A. Beneficial effect of hormone replacement therapy on weight loss in obese menopausal women. Maturitas. 1999 Aug 16;32(3):147-53. doi: 10.1016/s0378-5122(99)00037-7. PMID: 10515671.

12. Shiloah, Renata and Hamilton, Rainey and Vazquez, Liz, "Reversal of Risk for Metabolic Syndrome in a Post-Menopausal Woman Presenting With Multiple Medical Problems Using an Integrative Treatment Approach: A Case Report," (December 18, 2019). Available at SSRN: https://ssrn.com/abstract=3506037 or http://dx.-doi.org/10.2139/ssrn.3506037.

13. Stotland NL. Menopause: social expectations, women's realities. Arch Womens Ment Health. 2002 Aug;5(1):5-8. doi: 10.1007/s007370200016. PMID: 12503068.

14. Burger HG. Unpredictable endocrinology of the menopause transition: clinical, diagnostic and management implications. Menopause Int. 2011 Dec;17(4):153-4. doi: 10.1258/mi.2011.011026. Epub 2011 Nov 25. PMID: 22120939.

15. Santoro N, Epperson CN, Mathews SB. Menopausal Symptoms and Their Management. Endocrinol Metab Clin North Am. 2015 Sep;44(3):497-515. doi: 10.1016/j.ecl.2015.05.001. PMID: 26316239; PMCID: PMC4890704.

16. McElmurry BJ, Huddleston DS. Self-care and menopause: critical review of research. Health Care Women Int. 1991 Jan-Mar;12(1):15-26. doi: 10.1080/07399339109515923. PMID: 1989958.

17. Caputo J, Pavalko EK, Hardy MA. The Long-Term Effects of Caregiving on Women's Health and Mortality. J Marriage Fam. 2016 Oct;78(5):1382-1398. doi: 10.1111/jomf.12332. Epub 2016 Jul 26. PMID: 27795579; PMCID: PMC5079527.

4. YOU ARE NOT ALONE

1. Sivarajasingam V. Breaking the silence around the menopause. Br J Gen Pract. 2022 Mar 31;72(717):170. doi: 10.3399/bjgp22X719093. PMID: 35361589; PMCID: PMC8966928.

2. Naworska B, Brzęk A, Bąk-Sosnowska M. The Relationship between Health Status and Social Activity of Perimenopausal and Postmenopausal Women (Health Status and Social Relationships in Menopause). Int J Environ Res Public Health. 2020 Nov 12;17(22):8388. doi: 10.3390/ijerph17228388. PMID: 33198407; PMCID: PMC7696753.

3. Rolls K, Hansen M, Jackson D, Elliott D. How Health Care Professionals Use Social Media to Create Virtual Communities: An Integrative Review. J Med Internet Res. 2016

Jun 16;18(6):e166. doi: 10.2196/jmir.5312. PMID: 27328967; PMCID: PMC4933801.

5. WHAT YOU EAT MATTERS

1. Silva TR, Oppermann K, Reis FM, Spritzer PM. Nutrition in Menopausal Women: A Narrative Review. Nutrients. 2021 Jun 23;13(7):2149. doi: 10.3390/nu13072149. PMID: 34201460; PMCID: PMC8308420.
2. "Learning about Healthy Eating During Menopause," Alberta Health Services, accessed August 2, 2022, https://myhealth.alberta.ca/Health/aftercareinformation/pages/conditions.aspx?hwid=abk7408
3. Oldra CM, Benvegnú DM, Silva DRP, Wendt GW, Vieira AP. Relationships between depression and food intake in climacteric women. Climacteric. 2020 Oct;23(5):474-481. doi: 10.1080/13697137.2020.1736025. Epub 2020 Mar 17. PMID: 32180466.

6. HEALTHY EATING CASE STUDIES

1. Becker, S. L., & Manson, J. A. E. (n.d.). "Menopause, the gut microbiome, and weight gain: correlation or causation?" *Menopause: The Journal of The North American Menopause Society.* March 2021, Volume 28, Issue 3, p 327–331 doi: 10.1097/GME.0000000000001702. Retrieved November 21, 2021, from https://journals.lww.com/menopausejournal/Fulltext/2021/03000/Menopause,_the_gut_microbiome,_and_weight_-gain_.14.aspx?casa_token=_TTVbTdzPEk-AAAAA%3AQyMp_KO9kM-53YA8arXutFGfMgkk2JhFQXWy7Dd9Ee5nuFPkpAav-NinnhFCWrkekRs0bF095NTtG0sEeQoIPjSw.
2. Ibid.

7. RECIPES FOR RELIEF

1. Megan Ware, RDN, L.D., "Why Is Avocado Good for You?" Medical News Today, July 28, 2021, accessed August 2, 2022, https://www.medicalnewstoday.com/articles/270406#tips.

2. Fulgoni VL 3rd, Dreher M, Davenport AJ. "Avocado consumption is associated with better diet quality and nutrient intake, and lower metabolic syndrome risk in US adults: results from the National Health and Nutrition Examination Survey (NHANES) 2001–2008." Nutr J. 2013 Jan 2;12:1. doi: 10.1186/1475-2891-12-1. PMID: 23282226; PMCID: PMC3545982., https://pubmed.ncbi.nlm.nih.gov/23282226/.

3. Ibid.

4. David Railton, "What is the link between menopause and anxiety?", Medical News Today, May 3, 2022, accessed August 2, 2022, https://www.medicalnewstoday.com/articles/317552.

5. Kulkarni, S.K., Bhutani, M.K. & Bishnoi, M. Antidepressant activity of curcumin: involvement of serotonin and dopamine system. *Psychopharmacology* 201, 435 (2008). https://doi.org/10.1007/s00213-008-1300-y.

6. Hewlings, Susan J., and Douglas S. Kalman. 2017. "Curcumin: A Review of Its Effects on Human Health," *Foods* 6, no. 10: 92. https://doi.org/10.3390/foods6100092.

7. Grotto D, Zied E. The Standard American Diet and its relationship to the health status of Americans. Nutr Clin Pract. 2010 Dec;25(6):603-12. doi: 10.1177/0884533610386234. PMID: 21139124.

8. *Disclaimer: The hormone reset cleanse and lifestyle diet plan in this book is in no way to be used as a substitute for medications or medical advice prescribed by your medical doctor. If you are diabetic or have any chronic medical condition, please speak with your doctor before beginning these or any other changes to your diet. Please note that everyone is unique and may not experience the same relief at the same time.*

9. Mirdal, G. M. (2012). Mevlana Jalāl-ad-Dīn Rumi and Mindfulness. *Journal of Religion and Health, 51(4), 1202–1215. https://doi.org/10.1007/s10943-010-9430-z.*

8. MOVEMENT MATTERS

1. Grindler NM, Santoro NF. Menopause and exercise. Menopause. 2015 Dec;22(12):1351-8. doi: 10.1097/GME.0000000000000536. PMID: 26382311.

2. Jurdana M. Physical activity and cancer risk. Actual knowledge and possible biological mechanisms. Radiol Oncol. 2021 Jan 12;55(1):7-17. doi: 10.2478/raon-2020-0063. PMID: 33885236; PMCID: PMC7877262.

3. Voskuil DW, Monninkhof EM, Elias SG, Vlems FA, van Leeuwen FE; Task Force Physical Activity and Cancer. Physical activity and endometrial cancer risk, a systematic review of current evidence. Cancer Epidemiol Biomarkers Prev. 2007 Apr;16(4):639-48. doi: 10.1158/1055-9965.EPI-06-0742. PMID: 17416752.

4. Tabor E, Zagórski P, Martela K, Glinkowski W, Kuźniewicz R, Pluskiewicz W. The role of physical activity in early adulthood and middle-age on bone health after menopause in epidemiological population from Silesia Osteo Active Study. Int J Clin Pract. 2016 Oct;70(10):835-842. doi: 10.1111/ijcp.12874. Epub 2016 Sep 22. PMID: 27655014.

5. Dennis KE. Postmenopausal women and the health consequences of obesity. J Obstet Gynecol Neonatal Nurs. 2007 Sep-Oct;36(5):511-7; quiz 518-9. doi: 10.1111/j.1552-6909.2007.00180.x. PMID: 17880324.

6. Bernard P, Ninot G, Bernard PL, Picot MC, Jaussent A, Tallon G, Blain H. Effects of a six-month walking intervention on depression in inactive post-menopausal women: a randomized controlled trial. Aging Ment Health. 2015;19(6):485-92. doi: 10.1080/13607863.2014.948806. Epub 2014 Aug 18. PMID: 25133492.

9. YOGA & MEDITATION FOR MENOPAUSE

1. Vaze N, Joshi S. Yoga and menopausal transition. J Midlife Health. 2010 Jul;1(2):56-8. doi: 10.4103/0976-7800.76212. PMID: 21716773; PMCID: PMC3122509.

2. Ibid.

3. Banth S, Ardebil MD. Effectiveness of mindfulness meditation on pain and quality of life of patients with chronic low back pain. Int J Yoga. 2015 Jul-Dec;8(2):128-33. doi: 10.4103/0973-6131.158476. PMID: 26170592; PMCID: PMC4479890.

4. Biman S, Maharana S, Metri KG, Nagaratna R. Effects of yoga on stress, fatigue, musculoskeletal pain, and the quality of life among employees of diamond industry: A new approach in employee wellness. Work. 2021;70(2):521-529. doi: 10.3233/WOR-213589. PMID: 34633352.

5. Sengupta P. Health Impacts of Yoga and Pranayama: A State-of-the-Art Review. Int J Prev Med. 2012 Jul;3(7):444-58. PMID: 22891145; PMCID: PMC3415184.

6. Forseth B, Hunter SD. Range of Yoga Intensities From Savasana to Sweating: A Systematic Review. J Phys Act Health. 2020 Feb 1;17(2):242-249. doi: 10.1123/jpah.2019-0372. PMID: 31855852.

7. Zaccaro A, Piarulli A, Laurino M, Garbella E, Menicucci D, Neri B, Gemignani A. How Breath-Control Can Change Your Life: A Systematic Review on Psycho-Physiological Correlates of Slow Breathing. Front Hum Neurosci. 2018 Sep 7;12:353. doi: 10.3389/fnhum.2018.00353. PMID: 30245619; PMCID: PMC6137615.

8. Joshi S, Khandwe R, Bapat D, Deshmukh U. Effect of yoga on menopausal symptoms. Menopause Int. 2011 Sep;17(3):78-81. doi: 10.1258/mi.2011.011020. PMID: 21903710.

10. COMPLEMENTARY & ALTERNATIVE TREATMENTS (CAM)

1. Johnson A, Roberts L, Elkins G. Complementary and Alternative Medicine for Menopause. J Evid Based Integr Med. 2019 Jan-Dec;24:2515690X19829380. doi: 10.1177/2515690X19829380. PMID: 30868921; PMCID: PMC6419242.
2. Johnson A, Roberts L, Elkins G. Complementary and Alternative Medicine for Menopause. J Evid Based Integr Med. 2019 Jan-Dec;24:2515690X19829380. doi: 10.1177/2515690X19829380. PMID: 30868921; PMCID: PMC6419242.
3. Moore TR, Franks RB, Fox C. Review of Efficacy of Complementary and Alternative Medicine Treatments for Menopausal Symptoms. J Midwifery Womens Health. 2017 May;62(3):286-297. doi: 10.1111/jmwh.12628. Epub 2017 May 31. PMID: 28561959.
4. Dyer NL, Baldwin AL, Rand WL. A Large-Scale Effectiveness Trial of Reiki for Physical and Psychological Health. J Altern Complement Med. 2019 Dec;25(12):1156-1162. doi: 10.1089/acm.2019.0022. Epub 2019 Oct 22. PMID: 31638407.
5. Chase CR. The Geometry of Emotions: Using Chakra Acupuncture and 5-Phase Theory to Describe Personality Archetypes for Clinical Use. Med Acupunct. 2018 Aug 1;30(4):167-178. doi: 10.1089/acu.2018.1288. PMID: 30147818; PMCID: PMC6106753.
6. Ross CL. Energy Medicine: Current Status and Future Perspectives. Glob Adv Health Med. 2019 Feb 27;8:2164956119831221. doi: 10.1177/2164956119831221. Retraction in: Glob Adv Health Med. 2021 Apr 13;10:21649561211012196. PMID: 30834177; PMCID: PMC6396053.
7. Eckstein M, Mamaev I, Ditzen B, Sailer U. "Calming Effects of Touch in Human, Animal, and Robotic Interaction-

Scientific State-of-the-Art and Technical Advances." Front Psychiatry. 2020 Nov 4;11:555058. doi: 10.3389/fpsyt.2020.555058. PMID: 33329093; PMCID: PMC7672023.

8. Thrane S, Cohen SM. "Effect of Reiki therapy on pain and anxiety in adults: an in-depth literature review of randomized trials with effect size calculations." Pain Manag Nurs. 2014 Dec;15(4):897-908. doi: 10.1016/j.pmn.2013.07.008. Epub 2014 Feb 28. PMID: 24582620; PMCID: PMC4147026.

9. Chakras Energy Deficiency as One of the Cause of Menopause Symptoms in Women; Wei Ling Huang[*] Department of Infectious Diseases, Medical Acupuncture and Pain Management Clinic, Franca, Sao Paulo, Brazil.

10. Cho YJ, Sim KL, Cho SJ, Lee G, Jung IK, Yin C, Kim H, Lee JS, Ryu J, Kim WS, Shim I. Effectiveness of training program combining chakrayoga and meditation. J Complement Integr Med. 2019 Dec 21;17(1):/j/jcim.2019.17.issue-1/jcim-2018-0167/jcim-2018-0167.xml. doi: 10.1515/jcim-2018-0167. PMID: 31865288.

11. Dale C. *The Subtle body: An encyclopedia of your energetic anatomy.* Boulder, CO: Sounds True, Inc; 2009

12. Hill-Sakurai, L. E., Muller, J., & Thom, D. H. (2008). "Complementary and Alternative Medicine for Menopause: A Qualitative Analysis of Women's Decision Making." *Journal of General Internal Medicine, 23*(5), 619-622. https://doi.org/10.1007/s11606-008-0537-9

13. McManus DE. Reiki Is Better Than Placebo and Has Broad Potential as a Complementary Health Therapy. J Evid Based Complementary Altern Med. 2017 Oct;22(4):1051-1057. doi: 10.1177/2156587217728644. Epub 2017 Sep 5. PMID: 28874060; PMCID: PMC5871310.

14. "How to Use Reiki Principles to Boost Well-Being," Healthline, last reviewed August 20, 2020, accessed October 27, 2022, https://www.healthline.com/health/reiki-principles.

15. Choi J, Lee HW, Lee JA, Lim HJ, Lee MS. "Aromatherapy for managing menopausal symptoms: A protocol for systematic review and meta-analysis." Medicine (Baltimore). 2018 Feb; 97(6):e9792. doi: 10.1097/MD.0000000000009792. PMID: 29419673; PMCID: PMC5944692.

16. Nikjou R, Kazemzadeh R, Asadzadeh F, Fathi R, Mostafazadeh F. "The Effect of Lavender Aromatherapy on the Symptoms of Menopause." J Natl Med Assoc. 2018 Jun;110(3):265-269. doi: 10.1016/j.jnma.2017.06.010. Epub 2017 Aug 18. PMID: 29778129.

17. Soleimani M, Kashfi LS, Mirmohamadkhani M, Ghods AA. "The effect of aromatherapy with peppermint essential oil on anxiety of cardiac patients in emergency department: A placebo-controlled study." Complement Ther Clin Pract. 2022 Feb;46:101533. doi: 10.1016/j.ctcp.2022.101533. Epub 2022 Jan 5. PMID: 35007899.

www.ingramcontent.com/pod-product-compliance
Lightning Source LLC
Chambersburg PA
CBHW040134160726
48006CB00014B/1491